Children on the Move

Children on the Move

The Health of Refugee, Immigrant and Displaced Children

Special Issue Editor

Charles Oberg

MDPI • Basel • Beijing • Wuhan • Barcelona • Belgrade

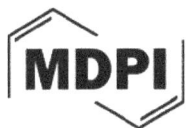

Special Issue Editor
Charles Oberg
University of Minnesota
USA

Editorial Office
MDPI
St. Alban-Anlage 66
4052 Basel, Switzerland

This is a reprint of articles from the Special Issue published online in the open access journal *Children* (ISSN 2227-9067) from 2018 to 2019 (available at: https://www.mdpi.com/journal/children/special_issues/healthcare_refugee_child).

For citation purposes, cite each article independently as indicated on the article page online and as indicated below:

LastName, A.A.; LastName, B.B.; LastName, C.C. Article Title. *Journal Name* **Year**, *Article Number*, Page Range.

ISBN 978-3-03928-200-5 (Pbk)
ISBN 978-3-03928-201-2 (PDF)

© 2020 by the authors. Articles in this book are Open Access and distributed under the Creative Commons Attribution (CC BY) license, which allows users to download, copy and build upon published articles, as long as the author and publisher are properly credited, which ensures maximum dissemination and a wider impact of our publications.

The book as a whole is distributed by MDPI under the terms and conditions of the Creative Commons license CC BY-NC-ND.

Contents

About the Special Issue Editor vii

Preface to "Children on the Move" ix

Charles Oberg
The Arc of Migration and the Impact on Children's Health and Well-Being: Forward to the Special Issue-Children on the Move
Reprinted from: *Children* **2019**, *6*, 100, doi:10.3390/children6090100 1

Stephanie Ettinger de Cuba, Allison Bovell-Ammon and Diana Becker Cutts
Constructing Invisible Walls through National and Global Policy
Reprinted from: *Children* **2019**, *6*, 83, doi:10.3390/children6070083 5

Nina K. Friedl and Oliver J. Muensterer
Special Aspects in Pediatric Surgical Inpatient Care of Refugee Children: A Comparative Cohort Study
Reprinted from: *Children* **2019**, *6*, 62, doi:10.3390/children6050062 10

Allison Bovell-Ammon, Stephanie Ettinger de Cuba, Sharon Coleman, Nayab Ahmad, Maureen M. Black, Deborah A. Frank, Eduardo Ochoa Jr. and Diana B. Cutts
Trends in Food Insecurity and SNAP Participation among Immigrant Families of U.S.-Born Young Children
Reprinted from: *Children* **2019**, *6*, 55, doi:10.3390/children6040055 18

Asterios Kampouras, Georgios Tzikos, Eustathios Partsanakis, Konstantinos Roukas, Stefanos Tsiamitros, Dimitrios Deligeorgakis, Elisavet Chorafa, Maria Schoina and Elias Iosifidis
Child Morbidity and Disease Burden in Refugee Camps in Mainland Greece
Reprinted from: *Children* **2019**, *6*, 46, doi:10.3390/children6030046 30

Andie (Saša) Buccitelli and Myriam Denov
Addressing Marginality and Exclusion: The Resettlement Experiences of War-Affected Young People in Quebec, Canada
Reprinted from: *Children* **2019**, *6*, 18, doi:10.3390/children6020018 38

Avinash K. Shetty
Infectious Diseases among Refugee Children
Reprinted from: *Children* **2019**, *6*, 129, doi:10.3390/children6120129 54

Eileen Crespo
The Importance of Oral Health in Immigrant and Refugee Children
Reprinted from: *Children* **2019**, *6*, 102, doi:10.3390/children6090102 75

Kathleen K. Miller, Calla R. Brown, Maura Shramko and Maria Veronica Svetaz
Applying Trauma-Informed Practices to the Care of Refugee and Immigrant Youth: 10 Clinical Pearls
Reprinted from: *Children* **2019**, *6*, 94, doi:10.3390/children6080094 81

Ziba Vaghri, Zoë Tessier and Christian Whalen
Refugee and Asylum-Seeking Children: Interrupted Child Development and Unfulfilled Child Rights
Reprinted from: *Children* **2019**, *6*, 120, doi:10.3390/children6110120 92

Melissa Diamond and Charles Oberg
Gender-Related Challenges in Educational Interventions with Syrian Refugee Parents of Trauma-Affected Children in Turkey
Reprinted from: *Children* **2019**, *6*, 110, doi:10.3390/children6100110 108

Logan DeBord, Kali Ann Hopkins and Padma Swamy
Challenges in Caring for Linguistic Minorities in the Pediatric Population
Reprinted from: *Children* **2019**, *6*, 87, doi:10.3390/children6080087 117

Ranit Mishori
The Use of Age Assessment in the Context of Child Migration: Imprecise, Inaccurate, Inconclusive and Endangers Children's Rights
Reprinted from: *Children* **2019**, *6*, 85, doi:10.3390/children6070085 121

Charles Oberg
The Rights of *Children on the Move* and the Budapest Declaration
Reprinted from: *Children* **2018**, *5*, 61, doi:10.3390/children5050061 126

About the Special Issue Editor

Charles Oberg is a Professor Emeritus at the University of Minnesota in pediatrics and public health, as well as the former Chief of pediatrics at Hennepin County Medical Center in Minneapolis, MN, USA. Dr. Oberg is an outspoken advocate for children's rights and the needs of vulnerable children. He is a renowned clinician, educator, and researcher who has dedicated his work to the care of immigrant, refugee and internally displaced children. He coordinates the International Society of Social Pediatrics and Child Health's (ISSOP) efforts to implement the Budapest Declaration on the Rights, Health & Well-Being of Children on the Move.

Globally Dr. Oberg has worked in Lesvos, Greece, providing needed medical care at the Moria refugee camp through the Netherland's Boat Refugee Foundation. In addition, he worked with Syrian refugees in a number of locations throughout northern Jordan, including the Al Zaatari Refugee Camp with the Syrian American Refugee Society (SAMS). Most recently, he helped to initiate a telehealth initiative between community health workers with physicians and hospitals in rural Tanzania with WellShare International.

Preface to "Children on the Move"

This Special Issue of *Children* will focus on the health of children experiencing migration as refugees or immigrants, and those internally displaced within their own country due to war and conflict. The explored topics will include adverse health conditions including the prevalence of specific infectious diseases, oral health and hospitalizations within refugee camps. It will also explore the mental health of children who have experienced significant trauma. It examines specific populations such as children with disabilities, unaccompanied minors and child separation at international borders. This Special Issue will also focus on the need to utilize best practice, trauma-informed care and care coordination. This includes the development of new clinical guidelines, the development of new care systems and advocacy for new policies addressing vulnerable children in need.

Charles Oberg
Special Issue Editor

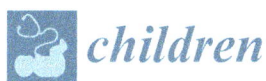

Editorial

The Arc of Migration and the Impact on Children's Health and Well-Being: Forward to the Special Issue-Children on the Move

Charles Oberg

Division of Epidemiology and Community Health and Division of Global Pediatrics, University of Minnesota, Minneapolis, MN 55455, USA; oberg001@umn.edu

Received: 1 September 2019; Accepted: 3 September 2019; Published: 6 September 2019

Abstract: Since the start of this millennium the diaspora of families with children has continued unabated. UNICEF estimates that nearly 31 million children have been forcibly displaced from their homes by the end of 2017. This includes 13 million child refugees, an estimated 17 million children internally displaced within their own countries and over 900 thousand children seeking asylum in a different country. Even more staggering is the 75 percent increase in the number of child refugees between 2010 and 2015. This Special Issue, Children on the Move: The Health of Refugee, Immigrant and Displaced Children, examines in detail the health and well-being of our most vulnerable children today. It follows the arc of migration from home country, through transit and finally the challenges experienced in a child's new country. The papers explore a variety of acute and chronic health conditions as well as the mental health of these children and youth. The articles examine the trauma experienced in their home country, the fleeing of war, violence and/or poverty, the travails during their journey, the stress throughout their stay in detention centers and refugee camps, and finally the transition to a new home country.

Keywords: children on the move; refugees; immigrants; trauma informed care; children's rights

---

Since the start of this millennium the diaspora of families with children has continued unabated. The general population's attention was drawn to the issue following the 2015 drowning of Alan Kurdi, the three-year-old Kurdish refugee from Syria. The photograph of the toddler lying face down on the shore made the journey palpable to millions worldwide. More recently, the image of children separated from their parents and held in detention centers on the southern border of the United States reawakened our collective awareness of the ongoing tragedy experienced by the global diaspora of families and their children.

UNICEF estimates that nearly 31 million children have been forcibly displaced from their homes by the end of 2017. This includes 13 million child refugees, an estimated 17 million children internally displaced within their own countries and over 900 thousand children seeking asylum in a different country [1]. Even more staggering is the 75 percent increase in the number of child refugees between 2010 and 2015 [2]. They are fleeing armed conflict, poverty, oppression and natural disasters, seeking to find a safe and welcoming new home.

This Special Issue, *Children on the Move: The Health of Refugee, Immigrant and Displaced Children*, examines in detail the health and well-being of our most vulnerable children today. It follows the arc of migration from home country, through transit and finally the challenges experienced in a child's new country. The articles examine the trauma experienced in their home country, the fleeing of war, violence and/or poverty, the travails during their journey, the stress throughout their stay in detention centers and refugee camps, and finally their transition to a new home country. It contains contributions from an international community of professionals working on behalf of all refugee, immigrant and displaced children. The papers explore a variety of acute and chronic health conditions as well as the mental health of these children and youth with an emphasis on trauma informed care. The contributions are grounded in the principles, standards and norms of child rights as articulated by the UN Convention on the Rights of the Child (CRC). All the articles provide new insights and strategies on how best to ground our clinical work as well as advocating for programmatic and policy change through a child rights based framework.

The Special Issue begins with an editorial by Stephanie Ettinger de Cuba, Allison Bovell-Ammon and Diana Becker Cutts that eloquently speaks to the "invisible walls" that are created through global policies within and across nations that first fail to address the antecedents of poverty, violence and climate change, and then isolationist and xenophobic polices that limit migration across borders. This is best exemplified by the present policy of the United States regarding its southern border and the especially harmful effect it is having on children and their families.

Nina Frield and Oliver Muensterer provide a glimpse into the hospitalization of refugee children admitted to hospitals in Germany. When families migrate from transitional refugee camps to hopefully their final destination, the morbidity and health burden frequently migrates with them. Their study is a retrospective review over a 10-year span. They found that hospitalized refugee children were significantly more likely to experience anemia, colonized with Methicillin-resistant *Staph aureus*, minor trauma, and esophageal foreign bodies as compared to non-refugee children. The results speak to the need to remain vigilant in the screening and assessment of refugee children once they have reached their destination.

Allison Bovell-Ammon, Stephanie Ettinger de Cuba, Sharon Coleman and colleagues provide an important paper from the Children's Healthwatch collaborative that highlights a worrying trend of increased food insecurity rates and decreased participation in the Supplemental Nutrition Assistance Program (SNAP) amongst children born in the United States to immigrant families. This investigation of economic and nutritional hardship complements the other articles in the Special Issue and completes the arc regarding the family diaspora over the last decade. Specifically, the ongoing stress that accompanies the migration of families from their country of origin to the assimilation to a new home. The findings have major policy implication for the United States' policies toward immigration and identifies that restrictive policies do have human consequences for children and youth.

Asterios Kampouras, Georgios Tzikos, Eustathios Partsanakis and colleagues examine the prevalence of disease and its resultant morbidity in the refugee camps on mainland Greece. A full 45% percent of those seen in the primary care office were infants, children and adolescents. The paper explores the magnitude of acute and chronic infectious diseases as well as non-communicable conditions including those associated with trauma and/or stress. The evolution in the approach to sheltering from a short-term way station into a long term encampment occurring during the winter months is poignant. It speaks to the adversity faced by these families as well as the need for policies by countries who are receiving migrating families with children.

The article by Andie Buccitelli and Myriam Denov explores the barriers experienced by young refugees fleeing war and conflict who are seeking asylum in Quebec, Canada. They face a myriad of care systems that are insensitive to their needs, values and beliefs. Trauma is a consistent and pervasive experience that spans from their home country, dangerous travels and resettlement at their destination. The paper examines a number of alternative approaches that were generated from the youths' insights. These approaches validate their own identity and lived experiences so as to facilitate adjustment to their new home now as well as their lives for the foreseeable future.

Eileen Crespo highlights in her review the importance of oral health for newly arrived children in the United States. For these new arrivals, oral health is often a significant issue, with the severity of dental disease varying by the country of origin as well as cultural beliefs that can hinder access to care. It concludes with a call to health care providers to recognize oral health problems, make appropriate referrals and communicate effectively with families on the need for both preventive oral health and care.

Kathleen Miller, Calla Brown, Maura Schramko and Maria Svetaz provide a review of trauma-informed care approaches designed to address the toxic stress and trauma experience by refugee youth. It outlines 10 clinical pearls that provides guidance to providers who are caring for this vulnerable group of children and youth. These included utilizing a strength-based approach to care, creating an immigrant-friendly environment that promotes trusting relations, and utilizing a two-generational approach to care and advocacy both within the clinic and community.

Logan DeBord, Kali Hopkins and Padma Swamy provide a unique insight from the trainee perspective on providing care for children on the move. They provide two case studies that highlight the need for quality interpreters/translators when working with refugee and immigrant families. They also provide recommendations on the need for medical education changes designed to address this issue.

Ranit Mishori provides an introduction to the topic of age assessment of minors crossing international borders and the difficulty of establishing the correct assessment of the age of immigrant and refugee children. This introduction provides a summary of the best practices presently available in estimating a child's chronological age. It discusses how medical knowledge can be misused during this sentinel event and concludes with a series of recommendations on adopting best policies, procedures and practices in the initial assessment and evaluation.

Ziba Vighri, Zoë Tessier and Christian Whalen, in recognition of the 30th anniversary of the UN Convention on the Rights of the Child (CRC), examine in depth the rights to provide for and protect children who have been displaced from their homes due to violence and war. The manuscript outlines the ramifications on children's health and development. It provides an in-depth analysis of the mandated provisions of the CRC dedicated to protecting displaced and asylum-seeking children.

Melissa Diamond and Charles Oberg provide a brief report on the trauma experience of Syrian refugee families and their children presently living in Turkey. It explores gender related trauma such as sexual violence, domestic violence and cultural constructions of masculinity, as well as the impact on the educational experience of Syrian children. The paper concludes with a call for increased integration of parent trauma support in educational intervention trainings and the creation of safe spaces where mothers and fathers can discuss their own trauma and in hope of enhancing educational program efficacy for their children.

Avinash Shetty provides a comprehensive review of infectious diseases experienced by refugee children. The review focuses on the notable infectious diseases of active tuberculosis, HIV, hepatitis B and C and malaria as well as other parasitic infections. It also highlights vaccine preventable diseases. It provides a summary of health assessment guidelines for newly arriving immigrant and refugee children.

The Special Issue concludes with an opinion piece by the Special Issue Guest Editor, Charles Oberg on the *Budapest Declaration*, summarizing this landmark document on the rights of immigrant and refugee children [3]. It also discusses how as child health providers we must alter our approaches to a holistic plan based on a child rights based approach (CRBA) that melds the intersection between health care, health systems, policies and programs [4]. It demands we advocate for a new approach in the 21st century to global migration and the health and well-being of children and youth who are on the move.

References

1. UNICEF. Child Displacement-UNICEF. Data: December 2018. Available online: https://data.unicef.org/topic/child-migration-and-displacement/displacement/ (accessed on 9 August 2019).
2. UNICEF. *Uprooted-The Growing Crisis for Refugee and Migrant Children*; UNICEF: New York, NY, USA, September 2016; p. 3.

3. Goldhagen, J.; Kadir, A.; Fouad, F.; Spencer, N.; Raman, S. The Budapest declaration for children and youth on the move. *Lancet Child Adolesc. Health* **2018**. [CrossRef]
4. Tobin, J. Beyond the supermarket shelf-using a rights based approach to addressing children's health needs. *Int. J. Child. Rights* **2006**, *14*, 275–306. [CrossRef]

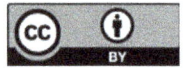

© 2019 by the author. Licensee MDPI, Basel, Switzerland. This article is an open access article distributed under the terms and conditions of the Creative Commons Attribution (CC BY) license (http://creativecommons.org/licenses/by/4.0/).

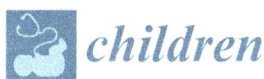

Editorial

Constructing Invisible Walls through National and Global Policy

Stephanie Ettinger de Cuba [1,*], Allison Bovell-Ammon [2] and Diana Becker Cutts [3]

1   Children's HealthWatch—Department of Pediatrics, Boston University School of Medicine, One Boston Medical Center Place, Vose Hall 5th floor, Boston, MA 02118, USA
2   Children's HealthWatch—Department of Pediatrics, Boston Medical Center, One Boston Medical Center Place, Vose Hall 4th floor, Boston, MA 02118, USA
3   Hennepin County Medical Center, Department of Pediatrics, G7, 701 Park Avenue, Minneapolis, MN 55415, USA
*   Correspondence: sedc@bu.edu

Received: 11 July 2019; Accepted: 15 July 2019; Published: 17 July 2019

Abstract: Worldwide 37,000 people are forced to flee their homes every day due to conflict and persecution. The factors that lead people to leave their home countries often originate with economic deprivation and violence, escalated to a level that becomes a struggle for survival. Climate change, as it has accelerated over the last three to four decades and negatively impacted natural resources, contributes to a parallel increase in strife and migration. The US response to migration has been to construct an "Invisible Wall" of isolationist and xenophobic policies, many of which are especially harmful to children and their families. The southern US border is perhaps the most high profile location of the Invisible Wall's construction, fortified by federal policies and a withdrawal from international cooperation. Global reengagement on climate change and migration, US ratification of the Convention on the Rights of the Child, and destruction of the Invisible Wall will help to create a world where children can thrive.

Keywords: climate change; migration; immigration policy; children's rights

Worldwide 37,000 people are forced to flee their homes every day due to conflict and persecution, according to the United Nations (UN) High Commissioner for Refugees [1]. The global levels of forcibly displaced people are the highest ever on record, numbering nearly 71 million people in turmoil from all corners of the globe, including Syria, Afghanistan, and South Sudan as well as Southeast Asia and Central and South America [1].

The factors that lead people to flee their home countries often originate with economic deprivation and violence, escalated to a level that becomes a struggle for survival. Whether the conflict is between ethnic or religious groups, law abiding citizens and gangs, or rival governments, many are rooted in a lack of equitable distribution of resources and an inability for people to generate income and wealth [2,3]. As competition for resources and power fans tension, scapegoats are sought, often fueling the blame of already historically oppressed groups [4]. Climate change, as it has accelerated over the last three to four decades and negatively impacted natural resources, contributes to a parallel increase in strife; Syria's civil war was sparked in part by a severe four-year drought causing 1.5 million people to migrate from rural areas to cities, increasing poverty and unrest[4]. In Central America, historical tensions over land ownership and rights were partially responsible for severe economic deprivation for large parts of the population and further exacerbated by US corporate and political involvement. Here, too, climate change plays a role. The "Central American Dry Corridor" is a zone that has been experiencing severe drought and floods, making it nearly impossible for families to earn a livelihood [5]. This extreme hardship fuels today's widespread violence and subsequent mass migration. In fact, the link between climate change and violence is now a demonstrated fact [6,7]. A systematic review of the global evidence found that collective violence and climate change, particularly when experienced as higher temperatures and extreme levels of precipitation, were repeatedly causally associated [7].

When climate change, economic deprivation, and violence come together, staying put becomes untenable, especially for parents and guardians desperate to provide for their children. Our research at Children's HealthWatch demonstrates over and over again that when parents lack the resources to provide basic needs for their children, they will go to great lengths of self-deprivation and personal sacrifice in order to protect their children from hardship [8]. The chance of a better future elsewhere, when there is none available otherwise, leads to a forced choice to risk all and flee. Each person's story of displacement is unique but all share fundamental characteristics—fear for their lives and livelihoods and the search for peace and stability [9]. With millions of people on the move, it is all too easy to get lost in the staggering numbers. The world was reminded again of the very human toll recently with the widely publicized photo of Óscar Alberto Martínez Ramírez and his toddler daughter, Valeria, face down in the Rio Grande after being swept away by the current when—his family unable to obtain an appointment for asylum with United States (US) authorities—they attempted to cross the river to the US [10]. This painful image reminded the world of the agonizingly similar photo of Alan Kurdi, half a globe away, whose drowned body washed up on the beaches of Turkey after his family attempted to sail to Greece for asylum.

What of such children? Are these sad images isolated cases or do they speak to more fundamental issues? According to the UN Office of the High Commissioner on Human Rights' Convention on the Rights of the Child, children are owed a special responsibility "by reason of (their) physical and mental immaturity, need special safeguards and care, including appropriate legal protection, before as well as after birth [11]." In addition, these special rights include those who are seeking refugee status—they should, "whether unaccompanied or accompanied by his or her parents or by any other person, receive appropriate protection and humanitarian assistance," including "protect(ing) and assist(ing) such a child and ... trac(ing) the parents or other members of the family of any refugee child in order to obtain information necessary for reunification with his or her family [11]." The United States has not lived up to this international code of responsibility—notably never ratifying the convention. Far from providing protection, humanitarian assistance, special safeguards, or assistance in reuniting families, the US government has made it official government policy to do the opposite. Reports from the southern border offer horrific stories of extreme neglect, unsanitary conditions, emotional and physical cruelty, and unnecessary and cruel family separation—all under orders from US Customs and Border Protection, which falls under the US Department of Homeland Security (DHS) [12,13]. Recent revelations of a secret Facebook group where Border Patrol members' racist and misogynist posts taunted migrants and officials in opposition to their actions and celebrated deaths and cruelty [14] were dismissed as "a couple of bad apples" by DHS' Acting Secretary [15]. However, with approximately 9500 members and Border Patrol leadership aware of the group for the past three years, that explanation defies credibility.

Beyond the present horrifying circumstances of the children and families, the harms being perpetrated are long-lasting and deep at both an individual and policy level. Neuroscientists from around the world have documented the fundamental and permanent brain changes that occur in children who have experienced upheaval, violence, and trauma, altering long-term socio-emotional well-being and ability to form attachments [16–21]. Their future, adult physical health is also threatened by significantly increased risk of poor cardiovascular health, acceleration of age-related disease onset, and early mortality [19,22]. These assaults on health put an entire generation of children at risk, digging a deeper hole of despair for their families.

Also disturbing is policy violence—a term referencing the effect of legislative, regulatory, and other types of policy decisions on people living in poverty [23]. The policy violence in place at the US southern border is part of a systematic effort to build an "Invisible Wall" [24]. The border is perhaps the most high profile location of its construction, but the source of its fortification includes policies that span DHS and the State Department to the Department of Housing and Urban Development, the Social Security Administration, the Department of Justice, and the Department of Agriculture. Federal agencies' explicit mandate from the White House has been to report on steps the agencies have taken to comply with laws restricting immigrants' eligibility for benefits, which benefits they administer are means-tested, and whether any other benefits they provide should be considered means-tested. Participation in means-tested programs have been proposed as a way to determine ineligibility for entry into the US and for adjustment of status once present (known as being a "public charge") [24,25]. These organized efforts, among others, are designed to make it dramatically more difficult for immigrants, refugees, and asylees to enter the country legally, extend a visa, receive assistance and be counted in the Census, apply for a 'green card' (Legal Permanent Residency), and apply for citizenship. The fundamental message being broadcast is "you are not welcome here." Given the zeal with which the changes are being applied to black and brown immigrants, it is an inescapable conclusion that racism and discrimination are powerful motivating forces [26,27].

At its core, these policy efforts are also a return to isolationism, a position that was rejected decades ago by world powers. This new embrace of isolationist, xenophobic stances, which have been supported by leaders in the US as well as other countries around the world [9], regresses us globally to a time that no longer exists, if such a time ever did. In fact, if we seek a world where children are able to thrive, the way forward can only be achieved in cooperation with others. The US once prided itself on its diplomatic place in the world as a partner and negotiator in multilateral efforts that helped bring peace. The professionalism of the diplomatic corps was revered and the US came to be seen as a moral authority. That position has crumbled with the withdrawal from international treaties like the Paris Climate Accord and mercurial stances on foreign and immigration policies.

An alternative approach, reengagement at the global level, is an opportunity to regain our footing and move toward real and lasting solutions of the twin challenges of our time—international migration and climate change. As leaders of small countries in the Pacific Islands have been teaching the world, the effect of climate change disproportionately places the greatest burden and cost on our world's poorest people [28], exacerbating global inequality [29]. Without collective effort, worsening conditions in poor countries will only spur further migration as heat increases crop failure, economic hardship, and violence. This fall, the UN will convene a global climate summit in New York. Other countries from Japan, to Germany, to the United Kingdom are making bold commitments to change [30]. If the US joined the fight, how much more progress could we make and how much more suffering could we avert—at home and abroad? Current US government policy calls on our darkest demons, but it does not have to be so—policy can be a force for dramatic and lasting good, creating a world where children can thrive. The US should reengage with the global community, finally ratify the Convention on the Rights of the Child, shoulder its share of responsibility to slow climate change and thus also migration pressures, immediately institute humanitarian standards for treatment of migrants, particularly children, and tear down the "Invisible Wall" [24].

References

1. Figures at a Glance—Statistical Yearbooks. United Nations High Commission for Refugees, 2019. Available online: https://www.unhcr.org/en-us/figures-at-a-glance.html (accessed on 10 July 2019).
2. Orellana López, A. Bolivia, 15 Years on from the Water War. 2015. Available online: https://democracyctr.org/article/bolivia-15-years-on-from-the-water-war/ (accessed on 10 July 2019).
3. Al-Jazeera. Syria's Civil War Explained from the Beginning: On March 15, the War Entered Its Eighth Year, 14 April 2019. Available online: https://www.aljazeera.com/news/2016/05/syria-civil-war-explained-160505084119966.html (accessed on 10 July 2019).
4. Batware, B. *Rwandan Ethnic Conflict: A Historical Look at Root Causes*; European Peace University: Stadtschlaining, Austria, 2012.

5. The Climate Reality Project. How the Climate Crisis Is Driving Central American Migration. 31 May 2019. Available online: https://www.climaterealityproject.org/blog/how-climate-crisis-driving-central-american-migration (accessed on 10 July 2019).
6. Miles-Novelo, A.; Anderson, C.A. Climate change and psychology: Effects of rapid global warming on violence and aggression. *Curr. Clim. Chang. Reports* **2019**, *5*, 36–46. [CrossRef]
7. Levy, B.S.; Sidel, V.W.; Patz, J.A. Climate change and collective violence. *Annu. Rev. Public Health* **2017**, *38*, 241–257. [CrossRef] [PubMed]
8. Frank, D.A.; Casey, P.H.; Black, M.M.; Rose-Jacobs, R.; Chilton, M.; Cutts, D.; March, E.; Heeren, T.; Coleman, S.; Ettinger de Cuba, S.; et al. Cumulative hardship and wellness of low-income, young children: Multisite surveillance study. *Pediatrics* **2010**, *125*, e1115–e1123. [CrossRef] [PubMed]
9. Sweetland Edwards, H. The Stories of Migrants Risking Everything for a Better Life. *Time Magazine*. 2019. Available online: https://time.com/longform/migrants/ (accessed on 10 July 2019).
10. Aguilera, J. How Controversy Over the Photo of a Drowned Migrant Father and Daughter Captured the Profound Cost of the Border Crisis. *Time Magazine*. 2019. Available online: https://time.com/5614807/photo-migrant-death-border-crisis/ (accessed on 10 July 2019).
11. Convention on the Rights of the Child. New York, NY, USA, 1989. Available online: https://www.ohchr.org/en/professionalinterest/pages/crc.aspx (accessed on 10 July 2019).
12. Fetters, A. The exceptional cruelty of a no-hugging policy. *Atlantic*. 2018. Available online: https://www.theatlantic.com/family/archive/2018/06/family-separation-no-hugging-policy/563294/ (accessed on 10 July 2019).
13. Raff, J. What a Pediatrician Saw Inside a Border Patrol Warehouse. *Atlantic*. 2019. Available online: https://www.theatlantic.com/politics/archive/2019/07/border-patrols-oversight-sick-migrant-children/593224/ (accessed on 10 July 2019).
14. Thompson, A.C. Inside the Secret Border Patrol Facebook Group Where Agents Joke About Migrant Deaths and Post Sexist Memes. *ProPublica*. 2019. Available online: https://www.propublica.org/article/secret-border-patrol-facebook-group-agents-joke-about-migrant-deaths-post-sexist-memes (accessed on 10 July 2019).
15. Acting Secretary McAleenan Appears on Fox News Channel to Discuss Crisis on the Border. Department of Homeland Security, 2019. Available online: https://www.dhs.gov/news/2019/07/05/acting-secretary-mcaleenan-appears-fox-news-channel-discuss-crisis-border (accessed on 10 July 2019).
16. Devakumar, D.; Birch, M.; Osrin, D.; Sondorp, E.; Wells, J.C.K. The intergenerational effects of war on the health of children. *BMC Medicine* **2014**, *12*, 57. [CrossRef] [PubMed]
17. Wright, M.O.; Master, A.S.; Hubbard, J.J. Long-Term Effects of Massive Trauma: Developmental and Psychobiological Perspectives. In *Developmental Perspectives on Trauma: Theory, Research, and Intervention*; Cicchetti, D., Toth, S.L., Eds.; University of Rochester Press: Rochester, NY, USA, 1997; pp. 181–225.
18. Macksoud, M.S.; Dyregrov, A.; Raundalen, M. Traumatic War Experiences and Their Effects on Children. In *International Handbook of Traumatic Stress Syndromes*; Wilson, J.P., Raphael, B., Eds.; Springer: Boston, MA, USA, 1993; pp. 625–633.
19. Locke, C.; Southwick, K.; McCloskey, L.; Fernández-Esquer, M. The psychological and medical sequelae of war in Central American refugee mothers and children. *Arch. Pediatr. Adolesc. Med.* **1996**, *150*, 822–828. [CrossRef] [PubMed]
20. Hoksbergen, R.; ter Laak, J.; Van Dijkum, C.; Rijk, S.; Rijk, K.; Stoutjesdijk, F. Posttraumatic stress disorder in adopted children from Romania. *Am. J. Orthopsychiatry* **2003**, *73*, 255–265. [CrossRef] [PubMed]
21. Goldstein, R.; Wampler, N.; Wise, P.H. War experiences and distress symptoms of Bosnian children. *Pediatrics* **1997**, *100*, 873–878. [CrossRef] [PubMed]
22. Ahmadi, N.; Hajsadeghi, F.; Mirshkarlo, H.B.; Budoff, M.; Yehuda, R.; Ebrahimi, R. Post-traumatic stress disorder, coronary atherosclerosis, and mortality. *Am. J. Cardiol.* **2011**, *108*, 29–33. [CrossRef] [PubMed]
23. Kaufmann, G. The Poor People's Campaign Calls Out 'Policy Violence'. *The Nation*. 2018. Available online: https://www.thenation.com/article/the-poor-peoples-campaign-calls-out-policy-violence/ (accessed on 10 July 2019).
24. Protecting Immigrant Families Campaign. 2019. Available online: https://protectingimmigrantfamilies.org/analysis-research/ (accessed on 10 July 2019).
25. Rose, J. Family Separations Under "Remain in Mexico" Policy. 2019. Available online: https://www.npr.org/2019/07/05/738860155/family-separations-under-remain-in-mexico-policy (accessed on 10 July 2019).

26. Farias, C. Is There Racist Intent Behind the Census Citizenship Question? *New Yorker*. 2019. Available online: https://www.newyorker.com/news/news-desk/is-there-racist-intent-behind-the-census-citizenship-question-wilbur-ross (accessed on 10 July 2019).
27. Understanding Trump's Muslim Ban. National Immigration Law Center, 2019. Available online: https://www.nilc.org/issues/immigration-enforcement/understanding-the-muslim-bans/ (accessed on 10 July 2019).
28. Worland, J. The Leaders of These Sinking Countries Are Fighting to Stop Climate Change. Here's What the Rest of the World Can Learn. *Time Magazine*. 2019. Available online: https://time.com/longform/sinking-islands-climate-change/ (accessed on 10 July 2019).
29. Worland, J. Climate Change Has Already Increased Global Inequality. It Will Only Get Worse. *Time Magazine*. 2019. Available online: https://time.com/5575523/climate-change-inequality/ (accessed on 10 July 2019).
30. Worland, J. U.N. Head: Climate Change Can Prove the Value of Collective Action. *Time Magazine*. 2019. Available online: https://time.com/5602482/antonio-guterres-climate-change-united-nations-summit/ (accessed on 10 July 2019).

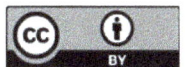

© 2019 by the authors. Licensee MDPI, Basel, Switzerland. This article is an open access article distributed under the terms and conditions of the Creative Commons Attribution (CC BY) license (http://creativecommons.org/licenses/by/4.0/).

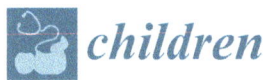

Article

Special Aspects in Pediatric Surgical Inpatient Care of Refugee Children: A Comparative Cohort Study

Nina K. Friedl and Oliver J. Muensterer *

Department of Pediatric Surgery, University Medical Center of the Johannes Gutenberg University Mainz, Langenbeckstrasse 1, 55131 Mainz, Germany; nina-friedl@gmx.de
* Correspondence: oliver.muensterer@unimedizin-mainz.de; Tel.: +49-6131-17-3865; Fax: +49-6131-17-6523

Received: 1 March 2019; Accepted: 28 April 2019; Published: 30 April 2019

Abstract: Background: Recently, the number of refugees in Germany has skyrocketed, leading to a marked increase in refugee children admitted to hospitals. This study describes the special characteristics encountered in pediatric surgical inpatient refugees compared to locally residing patients. Methods: Hospital records of minor refugees admitted to our department from 2005 up to and including 2015 were retrospectively reviewed. Demographic data, diagnoses, comorbidities, body mass indexes, hemoglobin values, and lengths of stay were extracted and statistically compared to local patients. Results: A total of 63 refugee children were analyzed and compared to 24,983 locally residing children. There was no difference in median body mass index (16.2 vs. 16.3, respectively, $p = 0.26$). However, refugee children had significantly lower hemoglobin values (11.95 vs. 12.79 g/dL, $p < 0.0001$) and were more likely to be colonized with methicillin-resistant *Staphylococcus. aureus* (8% vs. 0.04%, $p < 0.01$). Refugees were much more likely to present with burn injuries (16% versus 3% of admissions, $p < 0.001$), esophageal foreign bodies (4% vs. 0.5%, $p < 0.001$), as well as trauma, except for closed head injury. Conclusion: The cohort of refugee children in this study was found to be at a particular risk for suffering from burn injuries, trauma, foreign body aspirations, and anemia. Appropriate preventive measures and screening programs should be implemented accordingly.

Keywords: refugee; children; anemia; burns; trauma; foreign bodies; Methicillin-resistant *Staphylococcus aureus*; Multidrugresistant gram negative bacteria

---

1. Introduction

In the years 2014 and 2015, the number of incoming refugees in Germany skyrocketed. Approximately one-third of the arrivals were estimated to be minors [1,2], leading to a marked increase in refugee children admitted to pediatric and pediatric surgical departments. This wave has posed a variety of challenges to the healthcare system, ranging from language barriers and cultural issues to special resource allocation and funding of care [3].

We noticed that refugee children presented to our department with diagnoses and comorbidities that were markedly different than those of the native population. In particular, we were faced with a wave of burn and scald injuries at an intensity and scale not seen since the 1990s, before widespread anticipatory guidance and awareness campaigns were implemented in German society [4].

In this study, we investigated the special characteristics of refugee children admitted to a large academic pediatric surgical department in the southwest of Germany, focusing on diagnoses, colonization with resistant organisms, laboratory values, and growth parameters.

2. Materials and Methods

2.1. Ethics

The study was submitted to the ethics board of the state of Rhineland-Palatinate and deemed exempt from formal review due to the retrospective analysis of anonymous, routine medical data according to §36 and §37 of state hospital law.

2.2. Study Design

All patients admitted to our department from January 2005 until December 2015 were included. None were excluded. In order to discriminate between newly arrived refugee children and the local population, we stratified patient datasets by insurance status. While all children in Germany are generally insured either through private or publicly regulated companies, medical care of newly arrived refugees is funded by the municipality where the patient is registered. Once the asylum request is granted, which generally takes more than 6 months, the payer switches to one of the insurance companies. This difference is clearly marked in the electronic medical records, allowing us to discern between the newly arrived refugee children and those with permanent resident status.

Electronic medical records were then searched for demographic data, diagnostic and procedural codes, laboratory data, and findings of microbiological screening tests. These were statistically compared for differences between the cohorts.

2.3. Statistics

The statistical analysis was performed with SPSS for Windows 8, Version 22.0 (IBM Deutschland GmbH, Ehningen, Germany), using a t-test, Mann—Whitney test, and chi-squared analysis where appropriate. A level of $p < 0.05$ was defined as significant. Values are given as means with the standard deviation after the ± symbol, except when noted otherwise.

3. Results

3.1. Demographics

The annual numbers of refugee children admitted to our department increased at least 10-fold in the years 2014 and 2015 compared to the previous years from 2005 up to and including 2013 (Figure 1). A total of 63 admitted inpatient refugee children were analyzed and compared to 24,983 locally residing children. Many patients (69%) had no information on country of origin registered in the electronic medical records. The remainder came from Syria (11%), Albania (11%), Eritrea (8%), and Afghanistan (6%).

Refugee children were significantly younger (mean age 5.6 ± 4.7 years, median four years) than local residents (mean 7.5 ± 0.4 years, median 7 years, $p = 0.03$). Males were more prevalent in both groups (refugees 55%, locals 58%), without any statistical difference. There was also no difference in length of stay (median 4 days for both) between the cohorts.

3.2. Colonization

Screening for colonization with drug-resistant organisms was performed in 62% of refugees (40 out of 63 refugees). Those not screened were mainly presented before 2013, when universal screening was introduced in our institution. Screening was performed by nasal, axillary, and anal swab according to hospital policy, focusing on methicillin-resistant *Staphylococcus aureus* (MRSA) and multidrug resistant gram-negative microbes (MRGN). Overall, three refugee patients (8%) of those screened from 2013 onward were positive for MRSA, and only one patient of those screened from 2013 was positive for MRGN (2%). These ratios were markedly higher than for the locally residing population (0.04% and 0.06%, respectively, $p < 0.01$).

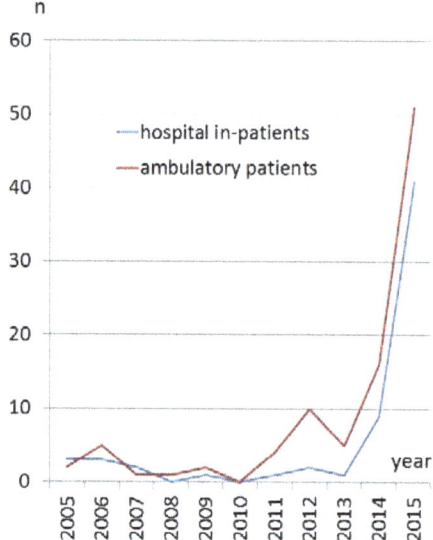

Figure 1. Number of refugee children treated at our department from January 2005 until December 2015. The blue line represents inpatients, the red line represents ambulatory patients. A sharp rise is evident in the years 2014 and 2015.

3.3. Growth Parameters

There were no differences between age-adjusted weight, height, or body mass index (BMI), except that the range and standard deviation of BMI was greater in refugees (Figure 2).

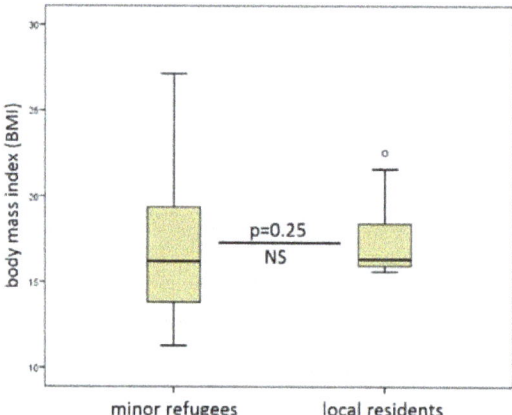

Figure 2. Comparison of body mass index (BMI) between refugees (left) and locally residing in-house patients. While the mean values were similar at 16.2 versus 16.3 ($p = 0.25$, nonsignificant (NS)), the range was greater in the minor refugee group.

3.4. Laboratory Parameters

As demonstrated in Figure 3, hemoglobin levels were significantly lower in the refugee cohort compared to the local population (mean 11.95 ± 0.9 g/dL versus mean 12.79 ± 0.8 g/dL, respectively, $p < 0.001$). Anemia, according to age-adjusted nomograms [4,5] was present in 16% of refugee children versus 3% of the locally resident inpatient population. No other differences in laboratory parameters were found.

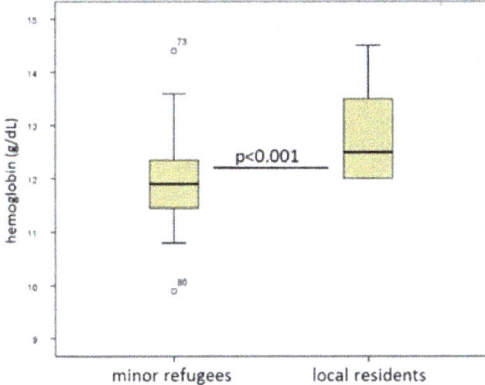

Figure 3. Hemoglobin values of refugee children (left) versus locally residing pediatric surgical inpatients (right). Refugees had significantly lower values and were more likely at risk for anemia.

3.5. Admission Diagnosis

There were clear differences in the rates of certain admission diagnoses recorded in the two cohorts (Figure 4). While locally residing patients were about 3 times more likely to be admitted with a closed head injury, refugee children were 5.5 times more likely to suffer burns, and 8 times more likely to have a retained esophageal foreign body or wrist injury. In addition, other trauma, such as kidney injury, ankle injury, and elbow fracture, was documented more often than compared the local population.

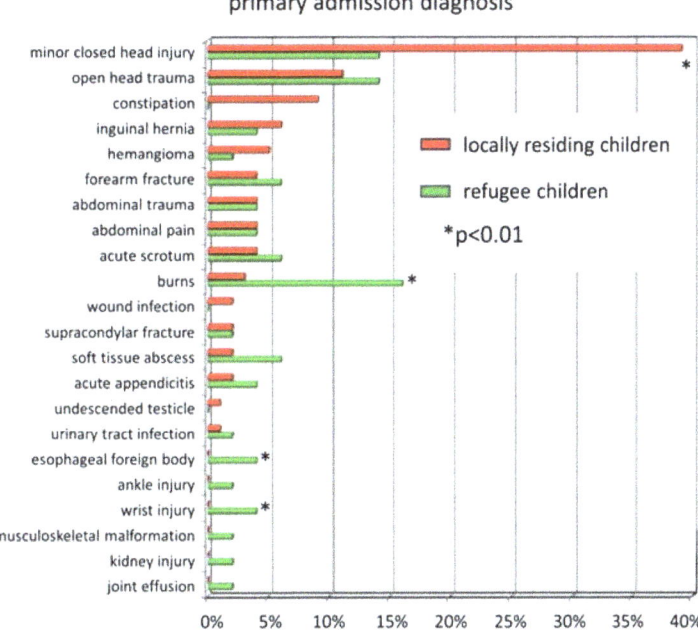

Figure 4. Relative proportion of admission diagnoses of refugee children (in green) and locally residing patients (in red) admitted to pediatric surgery from January 2005 until December 2015. While minor closed head injuries were more common in locals, refugees were more likely to be diagnosed with burns, esophageal foreign bodies, wrist injuries, and other types of trauma combined.

Concerning the burns, the most common mechanisms of injury were scald injuries. In about half of the cases, the child pulled down a pot, water boiler, or other form of container from a table or kitchen counter. The burn victims in the refugee cohort were 6 girls and 2 boys, with a combined median age of 3 years.

4. Discussion

Minors are a substantial portion of the refugee population around the world. In several reports, about one-third of refugees were below 18 years of age [6,7], and of those, around one-quarter were unaccompanied [8]. In the year 2015, immigration to Germany reached a peak of grossly over 2 million [9], and many of these immigrants were refugees that later applied for asylum. This wave of immigrants, who mainly originated from war-torn countries such as Syria and Afghanistan, presented a formidable challenge to the social and medical system in Germany. Most of the arrivals were initially housed in rapidly designated refugee facilities. By German law, before asylum status is granted, emergency medical care for refugees is covered by the municipality where the individual patient is accommodated, and this sometimes places an extreme economic burden and risk upon small towns and cities.

While there is an increasingly robust body of literature on the mental health of young refugees in Germany [10–13], other aspects of pediatric healthcare for refugees are less well-defined [14]. In addition, there is even less information on the surgical issues relevant to refugee children in Germany [15]. One report from Switzerland in 2015 found a high burden of infections in refugee children [16], and this was corroborated by a German study from 2016 [17]. Both studies describe the lack of systematic data on other health aspects, as well as challenges regarding legal conditions, language, and cultural competencies, and the underreporting of injuries. This is why we conducted our study on the special aspects of inpatient pediatric surgical care of minor refugees admitted over the course of 11 years, with a special focus on those that arrived during the last refugee wave during the years 2014 and 2015.

The care of this vulnerable population presents several challenges. Colonization with multidrug resistant organisms is a problem, since it requires isolation of the patient and thereby increases treatment complexity. In our study, refugee children were much more likely to be colonized than the general population. This is in line with other studies which have found similar results. In one study of 383 minor refugees at the University of Münster [18], 9.8% were colonized with MRSA, and 12.9% were colonized with MRGN. In a screening study of 119 unaccompanied minor refugees in Frankfurt [19], Enterobacteriaceae with extended spectrum beta-lactamases (ESBL) were found in 35% of cases. Higher numbers of MRGN (35%) colonization were found in a study from Mannheim [20], while MRSA colonization (7%) was similar to the rates in our population. The reasons for the higher risk of colonization with multidrug-resistant organisms are unclear, but most likely associated with the crowded living conditions in the shelter and suboptimal hygienic conditions. At this time, there is no study that has looked at overall exposure to antibiotics in refugee versus locally residing children.

Anemia is common in refugee children around the world [21–24]. This finding is most likely due to poor nutrition and iron deficiency, but other factors, such as vitamin deficiency [25], unrecognized metabolic conditions [26], infections, or hematologic disorders [27], may also play a role. Finally, the lower hemoglobin values may also reflect acute blood loss from trauma or chronic inflammation.

There are several possible causes that may explain the increased risk of refugee children suffering a burn, particularly scald injuries. Others have found a similar preponderance of burn injuries among refugee children [28]. Similarly, a Turkish pediatric hospital registered a high number of Syrian refugee children being treated from January 2016 to August 2017, with burn injury being one of the most common reasons for admission, after upper respiratory infection and gastroenteritis [29]. On the one hand, these children live in very tight conditions, in which several families use one kitchen to prepare tea or soup. In our study cohort, in one-half of the refugee children that suffered burn injuries, the mechanism was spilled hot tea or hot water for tea preparation. Additionally, in one-third of cases, the child or someone else had tripped over an electric cord that resulted in a spill of hot liquid over the child. An extensive systematic review on the epidemiology of burn injuries by Dissanaike and Rahimi corroborates our findings, in that there were strong sociocultural differences in the distribution of pediatric burn injuries, that scald injuries were the most common, and that over 50% of those injuries were associated with food preparation [30]. Hence, the crowded living space in a refugee shelter may predispose children to be in the kitchen while food is being cooked or water is being boiled. Many of the families come from cultures where hot tea is a preferred beverage. Additionally, some donated cooking equipment, including water heaters, toasters, samovars, electric grill ovens, and other items, may be old, out-of-date, or dysfunctional, and therefore not meet current safety standards. Finally, the refugee families may not have had the same exposure to child safety campaigns as the German population, in which the incidence and severity of burns has declined continuously over the last 25 years [4]. As a result, we would propose actively implementing regular burn prevention safety campaigns in all refugee shelters where children and families are accommodated.

Similar mechanisms may play a role in the relatively high incidence of esophageal foreign bodies found in our study. In the crammed environment of the refugee facilities, small objects may be left on the floor where infants and toddlers play. Most of these items are coins. However, the retention of button batteries in the esophagus may cause life-threatening complications. Thus, prevention campaigns should be implemented in refugee facilities on the dangers of leaving small objects, coins, and particularly button batteries accessible to small children.

Trauma, in general, was more common among refugee children than in the locally residing population, except for minor (in the sense of light, as opposed to severe) closed head injury. In order to understand our numbers, it must be said that in our environment, children with concussions and emesis after closed head injury are primarily admitted and observed in an effort to avoid a computed tomography of the head and the associated radiation exposure. Minor closed head trauma may not be perceived as a compelling reason to come to the hospital for evaluation by refugee families to the same extent as it is for resident parents, explaining the discrepancy observed.

Our study has several weaknesses. First, the overall number of refugee patients is limited, although the admission rates increased markedly over the last 2 years of the study interval. The mechanism of identification using payer information may have missed some children. Additionally, as there were local health clinics set up in the refugee camps by charity and volunteer organizations, only a select group of patients, most likely the more severely injured or ill, were most likely triaged to the hospital for inpatient evaluation and treatment. Refugees in general tend to use emergency care services less frequently than the general population [31]. In line with this finding, refugee children in Heidelberg, Germany, were admitted to the hospital 1.8 times more when they presented to an acute care clinic compared to the general population [32], indicating that there is a selection bias towards more serious pathology at presentation in minor refugees. Finally, the retrospective analysis of electronic patient charts may lack certain information that may be incomplete due to language and communication barriers.

Nevertheless, we believe that we evaluated a representative cohort of minor refugees that recently arrived in Germany because other pediatric surgical departments experienced similar findings, particularly regarding the high incidence of burn injuries.

In the German population, there is a relatively high level of consensus that minor refugees should have the same chances of access to education, social, and medical services as the general population [1]. In an effort to optimize the healthcare system of minor refugees, it is important to remember that the need arises spontaneously, depending on worldwide geopolitical events such as famine, drought, or war. Therefore, a general baseline preparedness must be combined with a commitment to spontaneous action [33]. It is our hope that the information presented in this study will contribute to the allocation of appropriate resources towards this vulnerable group.

5. Conclusions

Minor refugees in Germany have a higher risk of being anemic and being colonized by drug-resistant organisms than their peers in the local resident population. They also are more likely to suffer burn injuries and other types of significant trauma, other than minor closed head trauma. Care of these patients should focus on adequate iron intake, personal hygiene, antibiotic stewardship in the treatment of minor or viral infection to limit the emergence of drug-resistant nosocomial microbial flora, and safety measures to prevent trauma and burns. Furthermore, widespread MRSA eradication should be offered to families whose children screened positive for this. Education on how to prevent scalds and burns is particularly important in this context. We would strongly suggest implementing regular burn injury prevention and safety programs for all pediatric refugees and their families.

Author Contributions: Conceptualization, O.J.M.; Methodology, N.K.F. and O.J.M.; Validation, O.J.M. and N.K.F.; Formal Analysis, N.K.F.; Investigation, N.K.F.; Resources, O.J.M. and N.K.F.; Data Curation, N.K.F.; Writing—Original Draft Preparation, O.J.M.; Writing—Review and Editing, N.K.F.; Supervision, O.J.M.; Project Administration, O.J.M.; Funding Acquisition, O.J.M.

Conflicts of Interest: The authors declare no conflict of interest.

References

1. Plener, P.L.; Groschwitz, R.C.; Brahler, E.; Sukale, T.; Fegert, J.M. Unaccompanied refugee minors in Germany: Attitudes of the general population towards a vulnerable group. *Eur. Child Adolesc. Psychiatry* **2017**, *26*, 733–742. [CrossRef]
2. BAMF. Available online: http://www.bamf.de/SharedDocs/Anlagen/DE/Publikationen/Migrationsberichte/migrationsbericht-2015.html (accessed on 8 April 2019).
3. Nicolai, T.; Fuchs, O.; von Mutius, E. Caring for the Wave of Refugees in Munich. *N. Engl. J. Med.* **2015**, *373*, 1593–1595. [CrossRef] [PubMed]
4. Theodorou, P.; Xu, W.; Weinand, C.; Perbix, W.; Maegele, M.; Lefering, R.; Phan, T.Q.; Zinser, M.; Spilker, G. Incidence and treatment of burns: A twenty-year experience from a single center in Germany. *Burns* **2013**, *39*, 49–54. [CrossRef] [PubMed]
5. Beutler, E.; Waalen, J. The definition of anemia: What is the lower limit of normal of the blood hemoglobin concentration? *Blood* **2006**, *107*, 1747–1750. [CrossRef] [PubMed]
6. Mjones, S. Refugee children-a concern for European paediatricians. *Eur. J. Pediatr.* **2005**, *164*, 535–538. [CrossRef]
7. Lynch, M.A. Providing health care for refugee children and unaccompanied minors. *Med. Confl. Survi.* **2001**, *17*, 125–130. [CrossRef]
8. ISSOP Migration Working Group. ISSOP position statement on migrant child health. *Child Care Health Dev.* **2018**, *44*, 161–170. [CrossRef]
9. Statistisches Bundesamt. Migration 1991 to 2017. 2018. Available online: https://www.destatis.de/EN/FactsFigures/SocietyState/Population/Migration/Tables/MigrationForeignCitizensBetweenGermanyForeignCountries.html (accessed on 28 February 2019).
10. Buchmuller, T.; Lembcke, H.; Busch, J.; Kumsta, R.; Leyendecker, B. Exploring Mental Health Status and Syndrome Patterns Among Young Refugee Children in Germany. *Front. Psychiatry* **2018**, *9*, 212. [CrossRef]
11. Hodes, M.; Vasquez, M.M.; Anagnostopoulos, D.; Triantafyllou, K.; Abdelhady, D.; Weiss, K.; Koposov, R.; Cuhadaroglu, F.; Hebebrand, J.; Skokauskas, N. Refugees in Europe: national overviews from key countries with a special focus on child and adolescent mental health. *Eur. Child Adolesc. Psychiatry* **2018**, *27*, 389–399. [CrossRef]
12. Kim, S.Y.; Schwartz, S.J.; Perreira, K.M.; Juang, L.P. Culture's Influence on Stressors, Parental Socialization, and Developmental Processes in the Mental Health of Children of Immigrants. *Ann. Rev. Clin. Psychol.* **2018**, *14*, 343–370. [CrossRef]
13. Muller, L.R.F.; Buter, K.P.; Rosner, R.; Unterhitzenberger, J. Mental health and associated stress factors in accompanied and unaccompanied refugee minors resettled in Germany: A cross-sectional study. *Child Adolesc. Psychiatry Mental Health* **2019**. [CrossRef] [PubMed]
14. Kerbl, R.; Grois, N.; Popow, C.; Somekh, E.; Ehrich, J. Pediatric Healthcare for Refugee Minors in Europe: Steps for Better Insight and Appropriate Treatment. *J. Pediatr.* **2018**, *197*, 323–324.e2. [CrossRef]

15. Loucas, M.; Loucas, R.; Muensterer, O.J. Surgical Health Needs of Minor Refugees in Germany: A Cross-Sectional Study. *Eur. J. Pediatr. Surg.* **2018**, *28*, 60–66. [CrossRef]
16. Pohl, C.; Mack, I.; Schmitz, T.; Ritzh, N. The spectrum of care for pediatric refugees and asylum seekers at a tertiary health care facility in Switzerland in 2015. *Eur. J. Pediatr.* **2017**, *176*, 1681–1687. [CrossRef]
17. Spallek, J.; Tempes, J.; Ricksgers, H.; Marquardt, L.; Prüfer-Krämer, L.; Krämer, A. The health situation and health care needs of unaccompanied minor refugees—An approximation based on qualitative and quantitative studies from Bielefeld, Germany. *Bundesgesundheitsblatt Gesundheitsforschung Gesundheitsschutz* **2016**, *59*, 636–641. [CrossRef]
18. Kossow, A.; Stuhmer, B.; Schaumburg, F.; Becker, K.; Glatz, B.; Mollers, M.; Kampmeier, S.; Mellmann, A. High prevalence of MRSA and multi-resistant gram-negative bacteria in refugees admitted to the hospital-But no hint of transmission. *PloS one* **2018**, *13*, e0198103. [CrossRef]
19. Heudorf, U.; Krackhardt, B.; Karathana, M.; Kleinkauf, N.; Zinn, C. Multidrug-resistant bacteria in unaccompanied refugee minors arriving in Frankfurt am Main, Germany, October to November 2015. *Euro Surveill.* **2016**, *21*. [CrossRef]
20. Tenenbaum, T.; Becker, K.P.; Lange, B.; Martin, A.; Schafer, P.; Weichert, S.; Schroten, H. Prevalence of Multidrug-Resistant Organisms in Hospitalized Pediatric Refugees in an University Children's Hospital in Germany 2015-2016. *Infect. Control Hosp. Epidemiol.* **2016**, *37*, 1310–1314. [CrossRef] [PubMed]
21. Beukeboom, C.; Arya, N. Prevalence of Nutritional Deficiencies among Populations of Newly Arriving Government Assisted Refugee Children to Kitchener/Waterloo, Ontario, Canada. *J. Immigr. Minor. Health* **2018**, *20*, 1317–1323. [CrossRef]
22. Leidman, E.; Humphreys, A.; Greene Cramer, B.; Toroitich-Van Mil, L.; Wilkinson, C.; Narayan, A.; Bilukha, O. Acute Malnutrition and Anemia Among Rohingya Children in Kutupalong Camp, Bangladesh. *JAMA* **2018**, *319*, 1505–1506. [CrossRef]
23. Newman, K.; O'Donovan, K.; Bear, N.; Robertson, A.; Mutch, R.; Cherian, S. Nutritional assessment of resettled paediatric refugees in Western Australia. *J. Paediatr. Child Health* **2018**, *55*, 574–581. [CrossRef]
24. Pavlopoulou, I.D.; Tanaka, M.; Dikalioti, S.; Samoli, E.; Nisianakis, P.; Boleti, O.D.; Tsoumakas, K. Clinical and laboratory evaluation of new immigrant and refugee children arriving in Greece. *BMC Pediatr.* **2017**, *17*, 132. [CrossRef]
25. Mellin-Sanchez, L.; Sondheimer, N. An Infant Refugee with Anemia and Low Serum Vitamin B12. *Clin. Chem.* **2018**, *64*, 1567–1570. [CrossRef] [PubMed]
26. Schiergens, K.A.; Staudigl, M.; Borggraefe, I.; Maier, E.M. Neurological Sequelae due to Inborn Metabolic Diseases in Pediatric Refugees: Challenges in Treating the Untreated. *Neuropediatrics* **2018**, *49*, 363–368. [CrossRef] [PubMed]
27. Zur, B. Increase in genetically determined anemia as a result of migration in Germany. *Der. Internist.* **2016**, *57*, 444–451. [CrossRef]
28. Dempsey, M.P.; Orr, D.J. Are paediatric burns more common in asylum seekers? An analysis of paediatric burn admissions. *Burns* **2006**, *32*, 242–245. [CrossRef]
29. Güngör, A.; Çatak, A.I.; Çuhaci Çakir, B.; Öden Akman, A.; Karagöl, C.; Köksal, T.; Yakut, H.I. Evaluation of Syrian refugees who received inpatient treatment in a tertiary pediatric hospital in Turkey between January 2016 and August 2017. *Int. Health* **2018**, *10*, 371–375. [CrossRef]
30. Dissanaike, S.; Rahimi, M. Epidemiology of burn injuries: Highlighting cultural and sociao-demographic aspects. *Int. Rev. Psychiatry* **2009**, *21*, 505–511. [CrossRef] [PubMed]
31. Guess, M.A.; Tanabe, K.O.; Nelson, A.E.; Nguyen, S.; Hauck, F.R.; Scharf, R.J. Emergency Department and Primary Care Use by Refugees Compared to Non-refugee Controls. *J. Immigr. Minor. Health* **2018**. [CrossRef]
32. Lichtl, C.; Lutz, T.; Szecsenyi, J.; Bozorgmehr, K. Differences in the prevalence of hospitalizations and utilization of emergency outpatient services for ambulatory care sensitive conditions between asylum-seeking children and children of the general population: A cross-sectional medical records study (2015). *BMC Health Serv. Res.* **2017**, *17*, 731.
33. The, L. Migrant and refugee children need our actions now. *Lancet* **2016**, *388*, 1130.

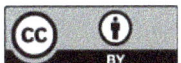

© 2019 by the authors. Licensee MDPI, Basel, Switzerland. This article is an open access article distributed under the terms and conditions of the Creative Commons Attribution (CC BY) license (http://creativecommons.org/licenses/by/4.0/).

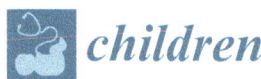

Article

Trends in Food Insecurity and SNAP Participation among Immigrant Families of U.S.-Born Young Children

Allison Bovell-Ammon [1,*], Stephanie Ettinger de Cuba [2], Sharon Coleman [3], Nayab Ahmad [1], Maureen M. Black [4,5], Deborah A. Frank [1,2], Eduardo Ochoa, Jr. [6] and Diana B. Cutts [7]

1. Boston Medical Center, Boston, MA 02118, USA; nayab.ahmad@bmc.org (N.A.); dafrank@bu.edu (D.A.F.)
2. Boston University School of Medicine, Boston, MA 02118, USA; sedc@bu.edu
3. Boston University School of Public Health, Boston, MA 02118, USA; Sharcole2@gmail.com
4. University of Maryland School of Medicine; Baltimore, MD 21201, USA; mblack@peds.umaryland.edu
5. Research Triangle Institute, Research Triangle Park, NC 12194, USA
6. University of Arkansas for Medical Sciences, Little Rock, AR 72205, USA; ochoaeduardor@uams.edu
7. Hennepin County Medical Center, Minneapolis, MN 55415, USA; diana.cutts@hcmed.org
* Correspondence: allison.bovell-ammon@bmc.org

Received: 4 March 2019; Accepted: 30 March 2019; Published: 4 April 2019

Abstract: Immigrant families are known to be at higher risk of food insecurity compared to non-immigrant families. Documented immigrants in the U.S. <5 years are ineligible for the Supplemental Nutrition Assistance Program (SNAP). Immigration enforcement, anti-immigrant rhetoric, and policies negatively targeting immigrants have increased in recent years. Anecdotal reports suggest immigrant families forgo assistance, even if eligible, related to fear of deportation or future ineligibility for citizenship. In the period of January 2007–June 2018, 37,570 caregivers of young children (ages 0–4) were interviewed in emergency rooms and primary care clinics in Boston, Baltimore, Philadelphia, Minneapolis, and Little Rock. Food insecurity was measured using the U.S. Department of Agriculture's Food Security Survey Module. Overall, 21.4% of mothers were immigrants, including 3.8% in the U.S. <5 years ("<5 years") and 17.64% ≥ 5 years ("5+ years"). SNAP participation among <5 years families increased in the period of 2007–2017 to 43% and declined in the first half of 2018 to 34.8%. For 5+ years families, SNAP participation increased to 44.7% in 2017 and decreased to 42.7% in 2018. SNAP decreases occurred concurrently with rising child food insecurity. Employment increased 2016–2018 among U.S.-born families and was stable among immigrant families. After steady increases in the prior 10 years, SNAP participation decreased in all immigrant families in 2018, but most markedly in more recent immigrants, while employment rates were unchanged.

Keywords: immigrant families; food insecurity; supplemental nutrition assistance program

1. Introduction

One-quarter of children in the United States (U.S.) under age 5 have at least one immigrant parent, with 93% of these children born in the U.S. [1]. Previous research has shown that infants and toddlers in low-income families with immigrant mothers are more likely to be born at a healthy weight, to be breastfed, to live in a two-parent home, and to have mothers who do not use tobacco, compared to children in low-income families with U.S.-born mothers [2]. Immigrant families, however, compared to non-immigrant families, disproportionately experience food insecurity, struggle to afford housing costs, and lack access to health care—all factors associated with adverse health outcomes [3,4].

Food insecurity, even if experienced at mild levels or temporarily, is associated with poor physical and mental health for children and adults regardless of nativity or immigration status [5–11]. As the severity of food insecurity increases to affect the quality and quantity of children's food, the health impacts of food insecurity on child health also worsen [12]. The Supplemental Nutrition Assistance Program (SNAP), the largest nutrition program in the U.S., is strongly associated with improved food security and positive health outcomes from the pre-natal period through early childhood and into adulthood [13,14].

SNAP is a means-test entitlement program that is available to all citizens and legally authorized families and individuals with incomes low enough to meet eligibility criteria. Families are often made aware of the program through community-based resource connections, and information about the program is widely available. In 2017, approximately two-thirds of people participating in SNAP were children, seniors, or persons with disabilities, and the average household income for SNAP participants was 63% of the U.S. federal poverty line [15]. Families and individuals participating in SNAP receive a monthly allotment of funds that are restricted for the sole purpose of purchasing uncooked foods to be prepared at home. SNAP cannot be used to purchase hot foods, alcoholic beverages, vitamins, cigarettes, household supplies, or other non-food items. These benefits are issued monthly on an electronic benefit transfer (EBT) card that the participant is able to use at authorized food retailers. In addition to reducing food insecurity, SNAP also promotes better nutrition. Every state in the U.S. operates SNAP nutrition education programming designed to teach participants about the benefits of healthy eating [16].

While all SNAP participants live in households with low incomes and therefore have higher rates of food insecurity than higher income households, several studies have documented the program's effectiveness in reducing food insecurity across levels of severity [13,14,17]. SNAP is also a countercyclical program, designed to expand during recessions when unemployment rates are high—as it did during the recent Great Recession, which began in December 2007 and officially ended in June 2009—and contract when unemployment rates are lower. Because of the countercyclical nature of SNAP, it is sensitive to trends in employment.

A large body of evidence documents the link between SNAP and child health. Mothers who participate in SNAP during pregnancy are more likely to have healthier babies compared to SNAP-eligible non-participants [18]. Young children in SNAP-participating families are less likely to be hospitalized, underweight, or at risk of developmental delays compared to SNAP-eligible non-participating families [19]. SNAP has also been shown to reduce food insecurity and poor health outcomes among children of all ages [20–22]. Even though SNAP effectively reduces food insecurity and improves health, it is underutilized, particularly by immigrant families. Federal regulations specify that documented immigrant adults who have been in the U.S. for less than five years are ineligible for SNAP, even if they meet all other eligibility criteria [23]. This is commonly known as the five-year bar. Although many families' U.S. citizen children may qualify for SNAP, research demonstrates that when parents are ineligible for assistance, their eligible children are less likely to participate in assistance programs [24]. Consequently, children of non-citizen parents are less likely to participate in SNAP. Because the benefits, when accessed, are often for the children only, mixed immigration status households have lower levels of SNAP benefits per household member when they do participate in SNAP and are at greater risk of food insecurity compared to households where parents and children are all citizens [25].

Over the past ten years, and particularly since 2016, increased immigration law enforcement, threatening anti-immigrant rhetoric, and public policy proposals that target immigrant families, including those that penalize immigrants for participating in assistance programs, have increased [26,27]. Anecdotal reports suggest that immigrant families may be forgoing participation in nutrition assistance and other federal assistance programs, even if eligible, due to fear of deportation or the negative effect of participation on their future U.S. immigration status [28,29].

We are unaware of any research that has systematically examined quantitative data comparing time trends in food security and SNAP participation among immigrant and non-immigrant families. This study aims to first document 10-year trends in household and child food security status and

SNAP participation among families with young children disaggregated by maternal nativity and, for mothers born outside of the U.S., tenure of U.S. residence. The secondary aim of this study, given the changes in the policy environment from 2016 to 2018, sought to understand trends in food security status, SNAP participation, employment, and demographic differences across these years. Changes in household employment among immigrant and non-immigrant families, which may explain changes in SNAP participation and food insecurity rates, were also examined.

2. Methods

Data come from the ongoing Children's HealthWatch study, a multisite cross-sectional study investigating associations between economic hardships, participation in assistance programs, and the health of young children and their families [30]. Caregivers of children under 48 months were recruited for survey participation by trained research assistants during their child's primary care appointment or emergency department visit in five U.S. cities (Baltimore, MA; Boston, MA; Minneapolis, MN; Little Rock, AR; Philadelphia, PA). Data for this study were collected between January 2007 and June 2018, a period encompassing the Great Recession and economic recovery. As previously published [31], eligibility included fluency in English, Spanish, or Somali (Minneapolis only), state residency, and knowledge of the child's household. Caregivers of critically ill or injured children were not approached, nor were those interviewed within the previous six months. Research assistants administered interviews to caregivers verbally face-to-face in private settings after gaining informed consent. Institutional review board approval was obtained at each site prior to data collection and was renewed annually.

Of 53,356 caregivers approached between January 2007 and June 2018, 5474 (10.3%) were ineligible for the study, and 4114 (8.6%) refused or were unable to complete the interview. To ensure that the sample included only families with some members likely to be eligible for SNAP, the sample was limited to children born in the U.S. with public or no health insurance. Of caregiver/child dyads who completed the interview, 354 (<1%) children born outside of the U.S. and 4342 (9.98%) children with private health insurance were excluded. Additionally, the sample excluded caregivers who completed the interview in Somali ($n = 168$), given the unique circumstances of Somali refugees in the U.S., who are more likely to be eligible for SNAP than other immigrant populations and to whom the five-year bar does not apply. The final analytic sample was 37,570 (Figure 1).

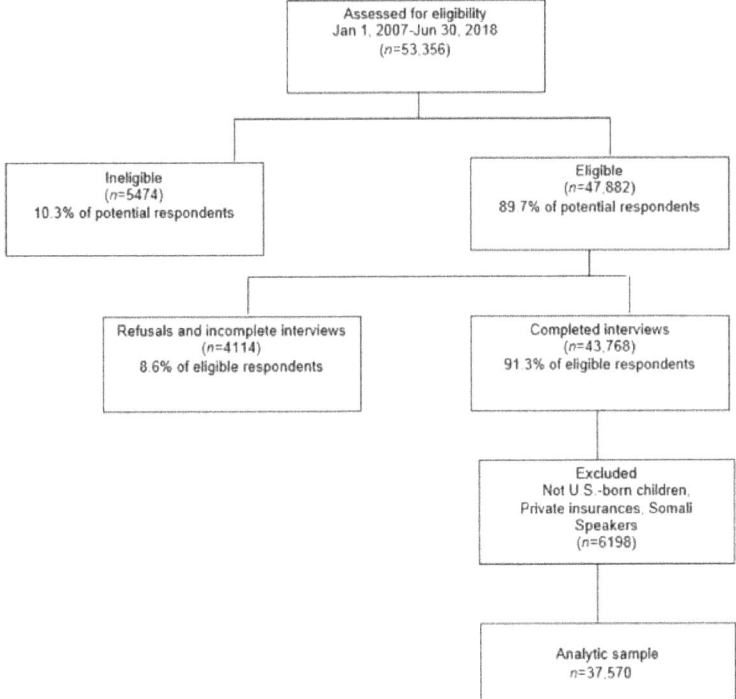

Figure 1. Description of analytic sample.

2.1. Independent Variables

2.1.1. Demographics

Caregivers reported the mother's age and race/ethnicity, their educational attainment, and their employment status. Child age was abstracted from medical records.

Mother's nativity and tenure in the U.S.: Caregivers were asked the birthplace of the biological mother and, if born outside of the U.S., the year the biological mother moved to the U.S. Of the caregivers interviewed, 93.7% were biological mothers. The sample was divided into three groups by nativity and tenure in the U.S.: (1) mothers born in the U.S. (U.S.-born group); (2) mothers born outside of the U.S. residing in the U.S. for five or more years (5+ years group); and (3) mothers born outside of the U.S. residing in the U.S. for less than five years, reflecting SNAP's five-year residency requirement (<5 years group).

2.1.2. Employment

Caregivers reported the number of employed members in the household. For this analysis, the variable was coded as any household employment vs. no household employment. Additionally, employment trends focused on the most recent years across the three groups—2016 through 2018. These years were selected in order to detect whether any change in food security or SNAP status in this period was plausibly related to increasing employment.

2.2. Dependent Variables

2.2.1. Food Insecurity

Household and child food insecurity were measured using the U.S. Household Food Security Survey Module (HFSSM). This survey module consists of 10 household-focused questions and eight child-specific questions assessing the previous 12 months. The HFSSM is the gold standard in the U.S. for assessing food insecurity. Households are considered food insecure if they report they are were unable to consistently afford enough food for all household members to lead active, healthy lives, and if this condition was a result of constrained resources. These analyses identified two levels of food insecurity: (1) household food insecurity (HFI)—three or more household-focused questions endorsed as sometimes true or often true vs. never true, but none on the child-specific scale; and (2) child food insecurity (CFI)—two or more child-specific questions endorsed as sometimes true or often true vs. never true.

2.2.2. SNAP Participation

Caregivers were asked whether their household participated in SNAP at the time of the interview.

2.3. Analysis

To examine the prevalence of household food insecurity, child food insecurity, and participation in SNAP stratified by maternal nativity and tenure in the U.S., we examined changes in each variable independently for each year over the study period, in addition to the 6 months from January–June 2018. In a secondary analysis, we analyzed changes in employment status between 2016–2018 stratified by maternal nativity and tenure in the U.S. Prevalence rates were compared across years through chi-square tests using a significance level of 0.05. All analyses were conducted using SAS software (version 9.3; SAS Institute, Cary, NC, U.S.).

3. Results

Overall, 78.6% of the households had U.S.-born mothers, 17.6% had immigrant mothers in the U.S. ≥5 years, and 3.8% had immigrant mothers in the U.S. <5 years.

The primary analysis found household food insecurity among all groups increased over the study period. Household food insecurity among the U.S.-born group increased from 8.7% in 2007 to 14.3% in the first half of 2018, reaching its highest point in 2014, with a prevalence of 16.1% ($p < 0.0001$). The 5+ years group experienced an increase in household food insecurity from 10.8% in 2007 to 25.0% in 2014, then a steady decrease to 12.6% by the first half of 2018 ($p < 0.0001$). Household food insecurity among the <5 years group increased from 9.9% in 2007 to 25.0% in 2013 and then declined to 10.6% in the first six months of 2018 ($p = 0.04$) (Figure 2).

Child food insecurity rates fluctuated among groups across the study period. Increasing from 6.7% in 2007 among the U.S.-born group, the prevalence in this group peaked at 12.7% in the first six months of 2018 ($p < 0.0001$). Child food insecurity rates for the 5+ years group increased from 17.2% in 2007 to 28.0% in 2010, then declined to 10.1% in 2018 ($p < 0.0001$). Child food insecurity was consistently highest among the <5 years group. In 2007, rates of child food insecurity were 25.2% among this group, increased to 33.9% in 2010, and then declined to 24.2% in the first half of 2018. The highest rate of child food insecurity among the <5 years group was in 2010 during the immediate aftermath of the recession, with a prevalence of 33.9%, declining over the next six years to 18.7% in 2017, though increasing again to 28.6% ($p = 0.035$) in the first half of 2018 (Figure 3).

SNAP participation varied across the groups and study years. Among the U.S.-born group, rates of SNAP participation increased from 57.2% in 2007 to 78.8% in 2013 and then steadily declined. SNAP participation among the 5+ years group was 30.8% in 2007, then rose to a high of 53.3% in 2013 before steadily decreasing to 42.7% in the first half of 2018. In the <5 years group, SNAP participation increased from 25.4% in 2007, to 48.9% by 2013, decreased to 43.0% in 2017 and then further decreased to 34.8% in the first half of 2018. All differences are significant at $p < 0.0001$ (Figure 4).

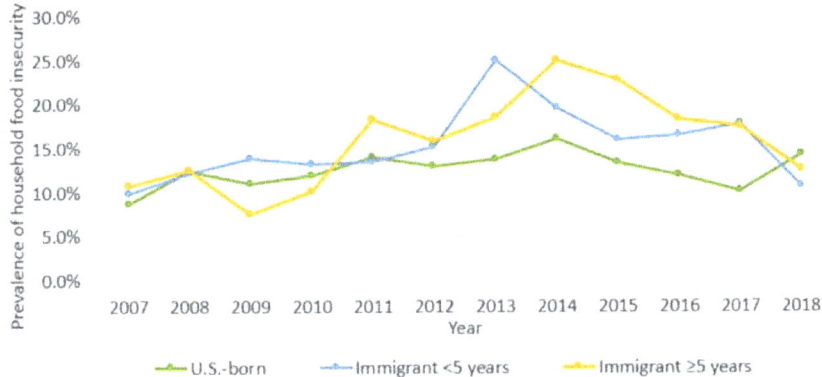

Figure 2. Trends in household food insecurity 2007–2018 by mother's place of birth.

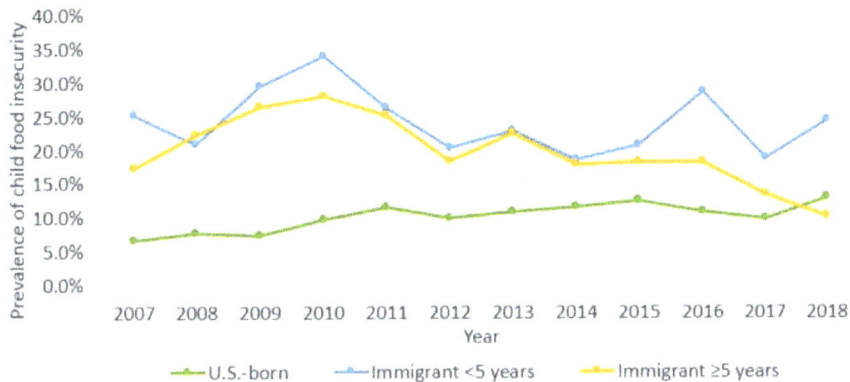

Figure 3. Trends in child food insecurity 2007–2018 by mother's place of birth.

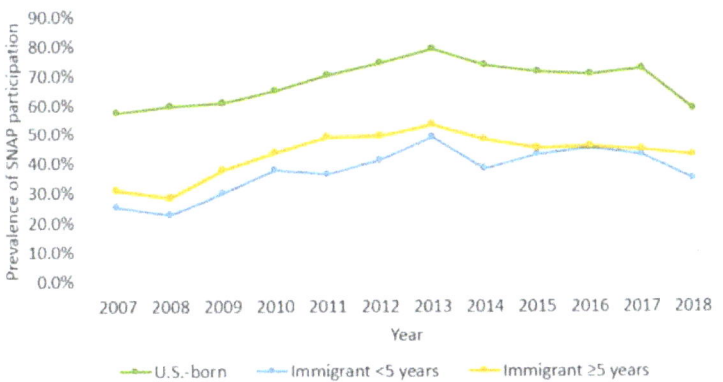

Figure 4. Trends in SNAP participation 2007–2018 by mother's place of birth.

The secondary analysis found differences in demographics and employment, which varied across groups from 2016 to 2018. Among U.S.-born mothers, there were demographic changes in the sample between 2016 and 2018. In 2016, 17.1% of mothers were White compared to 29.6% in 2018. There were also fewer Hispanic mothers and Black mothers in 2018 compared to 2016 (21.8% vs. 20.2% and 58.3% vs. 46.4% respectively) ($p < 0.0001$). The average age of U.S.-born mothers in 2016 was 26.6 (SD 5.3) and 27.3 (SD 5.5) in 2018 ($p = 0.0004$). The average age of the child was 19.2 months (SD 13.5) and did not vary across years. Caregivers in these families also had higher rates of education in 2018 than 2016, with 46.3% reporting having completed education beyond high school compared to 39.2% in 2016 ($p < 0.0001$); additionally, there were higher rates of being married/partnered in 2018 compared to 2016 (26.1% vs. 19%, respectively).

Among families in the 5+ years group, there were no demographic differences from 2016 to 2018. Across all three years, 73.5% of mothers were Hispanic, 21.2% Black, and 0.9% White. On average, mothers were 31.8 years old (SD 6.5) and children were 20.1 months (SD 14.3) old. One-quarter of caregivers (24.9%) had education beyond high school, and 43.5% were married or partnered. Among the <5 years group, on average from 2016 to 2018, 77.9% of mothers were Hispanic, 18.7% Black, and 0.8% White, which did not vary across years. The mean age of mothers was 28.7 (SD 6.5) years old across all three years. Child's age was the only demographic variable that changed significantly from 2016 to 2018 (12.9 (SD 11.9) vs. 18.3 (SD 12.9) months, respectively). Within this group, 34.6% of caregivers reported education beyond high school, and 40.2% were married or partnered, which did not vary by year (Table 1).

Analysis of employment trends from 2016–2018 also showed differences in employment rates across groups. Among U.S.-born mothers, household employment status increased from 78.3% in 2016 to 81.4% in 2018 ($p = 0.0014$). Household employment rates were, on average, 91% in the 5+ years group and 85.9% among families in the <5 years group, with no significant changes from 2016–2018 (Table 1).

Table 1. Demographics for 2016 to 2018 by mother's nativity and tenure in the U.S.

Question	Response	Overall	2016	2017	2018	p-Value
		U.S.-Born Mothers				
Mother Age	N	5132	2266	1538	1328	0.0004
	Mean (Std Dev)	26.8 (5.5)	26.6 (5.3)	26.8 (5.6)	27.3 (5.5)	
Child Age (Months)	N	5189	2287	1555	1347	
	Mean (Std Dev)	19.2 (13.5)	19.4 (13.7)	18.6 (13.3)	19.6 (13.4)	0.1207
Mother's Race/Ethnicity	Hispanic	1208 (23.6%)	492 (21.8%)	446 (29.2%)	270 (20.2%)	<0.0001
	Black|Non-Hispanic	2770 (54.1%)	1314 (58.3%)	837 (54.8%)	619 (46.4%)	
	White|Non-Hispanic	981 (19.2%)	386 (17.1%)	200 (13.1%)	395 (29.6%)	
	Other	158 (3.1%)	63 (2.8%)	45 (2.9%)	50 (3.7%)	
Caregiver Married/Partnered	Yes	1036 (20.0%)	434 (19.0%)	251 (16.2%)	351 (26.1%)	<0.0001
Caregiver Education	Less than high school	853 (16.5%)	382 (16.7%)	275 (17.7%)	196 (14.6%)	<0.0001
	High school	2231 (43.0%)	1009 (44.1%)	694 (44.7%)	528 (39.2%)	
	More than high school	2101 (40.5%)	895 (39.2%)	583 (37.6%)	623 (46.3%)	
Any Employment in household	Yes	4019 (78.4%)	1773 (78.3%)	1160 (75.8%)	1086 (81.4%)	0.0014

Table 1. Cont.

Question	Response	Overall	2016	2017	2018	p-Value
Immigrant Mothers ≥5 Years [a]						
Mother Age	N	1297	530	481	286	
	Mean (Std Dev)	31.8 (6.5)	31.6 (6.4)	31.7 (6.4)	32.1 (6.7)	0.5691
Child Age (Months)	N	1297	530	481	286	
	Mean (Std Dev)	20.1 (14.3)	20.7 (14.6)	19.6 (14.0)	19.8 (14.4)	0.3960
Mother Ethnicity	Hispanic	950 (73.5%)	398 (75.2%)	352 (73.8%)	200 (69.9%)	0.7082
	Black|Non-Hispanic	287 (22.2%)	112 (21.2%)	104 (21.8%)	71 (24.8%)	
	White|Non-Hispanic	12 (0.9%)	3 (0.6%)	5 (1.0%)	4 (1.4%)	
	Other	43 (3.3%)	16 (3.0%)	16 (3.4%)	11 (3.8%)	
Caregiver Married/Partnered	Yes	563 (43.5%)	230 (43.6%)	208 (43.2%)	125 (43.9%)	0.9858
Caregiver Education	Less than high school	485 (37.4%)	202 (38.1%)	191 (39.7%)	92 (32.2%)	0.1215
	High school	489 (37.7%)	207 (39.1%)	164 (34.1%)	118 (41.3%)	
	More than high school	91 (34.6%)	29 (31.9%)	40 (37.7%)	22 (33.3%)	
Any Employment in Household	Yes	1175 (91.0%)	474 (89.8%)	439 (92.0%)	262 (91.6%)	0.4222
Immigrant Mothers <5 Years [b]						
Mother Age	N	264	91	107	66	
	Mean (Std Dev)	28.7 (6.5)	27.9 (6.3)	30.0 (6.6)	27.8 (6.3)	0.0293
Child Age (Months)	N	264	91	107	66	
	Mean (Std Dev)	14.4 (12.1)	12.9 (11.9)	13.2 (11.3)	18.3 (12.9)	0.0095
Mother Ethnicity	Hispanic	204 (77.9%)	72 (80.0%)	85 (79.4%)	47 (72.3%)	0.4806
	Black|Non-Hispanic	49 (18.7%)	13 (14.4%)	19 (17.8%)	17 (26.2%)	
	White|Non-Hispanic	2 (0.8%)	1 (1.1%)	1 (0.9%)	0 (0.0%)	
	Other	7 (2.7%)	4 (4.4%)	2 (1.9%)	1 (1.5%)	
Caregiver Married/Partnered	Yes	106 (40.2%)	39 (42.9%)	44 (41.1%)	23 (34.8%)	0.5794
Caregiver Education	Less than high school	91 (34.6%)	32 (35.2%)	36 (34.0%)	23 (34.8%)	0.9208
	High school	81 (30.8%)	30 (33.0%)	30 (28.3%)	21 (31.8%)	
	More than high school	91 (34.6%)	29 (31.9%)	40 (37.7%)	22 (33.3%)	
Any Employment in Household	Yes	225 (85.9%)	79 (86.8%)	89 (84.8%)	57 (86.4%)	0.9111

[a] Immigrant Mothers ≥5 years: Families with mothers who immigrated to the U.S. more than or equal to five years ago. [b] Immigrant Mothers <5 years: Families with mothers who immigrated to the U.S. less than five years ago.

4. Discussion

During the Great Recession from 2007 to 2009, food insecurity increased for families with young children across all three groups. Families with immigrant mothers, in particular, had higher rates of household and child food insecurity during the height of the recession and a slower recovery than families with U.S.-born mothers. SNAP participation also increased across all groups between 2007 and 2013 during the Great Recession and its aftermath and then began to decline However, among families with U.S.-born mothers and immigrant mothers in the U.S. <5 years, there was a sharp decrease in SNAP participation between 2017 and the first half of 2018. However, small cell sizes for the first 6 months of 2018 should be interpreted with caution.

While an improving economy with higher employment rates might be a plausible explanation for this sharp decrease in participation in SNAP, employment trends varied only for the families with U.S.-born mothers while remaining constant for families with immigrant mothers in the U.S. <5 years.

The decrease in SNAP participation occurring concurrently with both an increase in employment and an increase in food insecurity among families with U.S.-born mothers may reflect a previously documented phenomenon where families whose SNAP benefits are cut off due to increased earnings experience a net loss of family resources placing them at higher risk of food insecurity [32]. The consistency of employment across 2016–2018 occurring concurrently with a decline in SNAP benefits among families with immigrant mothers who have resided in the U.S. <5 years, however, suggests that other factors may be contributing to this trend. The decline in participation among these families may be reflective of recent anecdotal reports suggesting that immigrant families are dis-enrolling or declining to enroll in federal assistance programs, including SNAP, out of fear of deportation or deleterious impacts on their future U.S. immigration status [29,33,34]. Other reasons for the decline in participation may be associated with this trend. Further research, however, is needed to discern the cause of the decrease. Qualitative methods that provide opportunities for immigrant mothers to respond to open-ended questions pertaining to their experiences in the U.S. and the reasons why they choose to participate or not participate in federal assistance programs such as SNAP may offer greater insights into the trends identified through this study. Research utilizing administrative data may also be able to examine nationally representative trends and potentially uncover other reasons for declining participating, such as disproportionate terminations or denials.

Several limitations of this analysis should be considered. The data come from cross-sectional sampling and therefore demonstrate associations, not causation. Due to only 6 months of available data for 2018, the cell sizes for this time period are small and therefore should be interpreted cautiously. All outcomes were self-reported, which creates a potential for bias in food security status and over- or underreporting of SNAP participation. Given that the current study includes only unadjusted outcomes, more research is necessary to examine associations adjusted for contextual factors that may relate to food security or SNAP participation. Further, the immigration status for the mothers, which impacts eligibility for SNAP, is unknown. The current policy context, however, makes these preliminary findings timely, and provides important evidence for ongoing policy discussions as well as directions for future research.

Policy proposals, such as the recent regulatory proposal to change the definition of public charge, may have contributed to this trend. Beginning in February of 2017, the federal administration began discussing changes to public charge, which is a term used by U.S. immigration officials to refer to persons who are considered primarily dependent on the government for subsistence. Immigrants subject to this consideration who are found to be or likely to become a public charge may be denied admission to the U.S. or denied adjustment to legal permanent resident status. To date, public charge determination has been limited to receipt of public cash assistance or institutionalization for long-term care at the government's expense.

Data in this study suggest a declining trend in SNAP participation among immigrant families, even as their employment remains constant and child food insecurity continues at a rate higher than the U.S.-born population. If the definition of public charge were expanded, as currently proposed by the present administration, to include participation in SNAP and potentially other supports like housing subsidies and Medicaid (public health insurance), rates of food insecurity among citizen children under the age of four years are likely to increase, along with associated health consequences [35,36]. Anecdotal stories from physicians, social service providers, and members of the community already describe fear among immigrant families related to participation in SNAP. A change to public charge could sharply increase this phenomenon in the short term.

Given the immediate and long-term health implications of food insecurity, especially child food insecurity [12], policy proposals that change public charge determination rules or impede SNAP participation among immigrant families of U.S. citizen infants and toddlers could have long-term negative consequences on public health and the health care system [37,38]. Beyond public policy change, it is important to increase education efforts among non-governmental, community-based organizations working with immigrant communities to inform immigrant families of their eligibility for SNAP and provide resources to local organizations that support enrollment in SNAP and other programs. In addition, ensuring data confidentiality for those applying for benefits, eliminating hostile anti-immigrant rhetoric in national discourse, and reducing barriers to nutrition assistance for families with low incomes regardless of parental nativity or immigration status [39] may benefit the health, growth, and development of the youngest citizens of the U.S. Future research is necessary to examine the sequelae of health outcomes associated with the trends documented in this study and identify potential solutions to remediate these trends. Further, as leaders in other countries outside of the U.S. propose policies that negatively target immigrants, research would be important to discern the potential ripple effects on the health of children and their families in those settings.

5. Conclusions

Over the last ten years, household food insecurity doubled for families with recently arrived immigrant mothers and their U.S.-born children while rates of child food insecurity remained alarmingly high. SNAP participation for these families decreased between 2017 and the first half of 2018, despite a lack of change in household employment status. These trends may be reflective of anecdotal reports in recent years that immigrant families fear participation in health-promoting nutrition assistance programs for which they may be eligible, including SNAP, because of fears of deportation or effects on their future immigration status. Policies that increase, rather than decrease, support for immigrant families with infants and toddlers may be necessary for reversing these trends that threaten the health and development of young children and their families.

Author Contributions: A.B.-A., S.E.d.C. and D.D.C. supervised data collection at the Boston site, conceptualized and designed the study, interpreted the analyses, and drafted and revised the manuscript. S.C. helped conceptualize and design the study, conducted the analysis, provided statistical expertise, and critically reviewed and revised the manuscript. D.A.F., M.M.B. and E.O.J. supervised data collection in their sites, helped conceptualize and design the study, and reviewed and revised the manuscript. N.A. critically reviewed and revised the manuscript.

Funding: This research was funded by the Annie E. Casey Foundation.

Conflicts of Interest: The authors declare no conflict of interest.

References

1. Children in U.S. Immigrant Families. Available online: https://www.migrationpolicy.org/programs/data-hub/charts/children-immigrant-families (accessed on 25 February 2019).
2. Chilton, M.; Black, M.M.; Berkowitz, C.; Casey, P.H.; Cook, J.; Cutts, D.; Jacobs, R.R.; Heeren, T.; Ettinger de Cuba, S.; Coleman, S.; et al. Food insecurity and risk of poor health among US-born children of immigrants. *Am. J. Public Health* **2009**, *99*, 556–562. [CrossRef] [PubMed]
3. Capps, R. *Hardship among Children of Immigrants: Findings from the National Survey of America's Families*; The Urban Institute: Washington, DC, USA, 2001.
4. Hernandez, D.J.; College, H.; Napierala, J.S. *Children in Immigrant Families: Essential to America's Future*; The Foundation for Child Development: New York, NY, USA, 2012.
5. Rose-Jacobs, R.; Black, M.M.; Casey, P.H.; Cook, J.; Cutts, D.; Chilton, M.; Heeren, T.; Levenson, S.M.; Meyers, A.F.; Frank, D.A. Household food insecurity: Associations with at-risk infant and toddler development. *Pediatrics* **2009**, *121*, 65–72. [CrossRef] [PubMed]
6. Shankar, P.; Chung, R.; Frank, D.A. Association of food Insecurity with children's behavioral, emotional, and academic outcomes: A systematic review. *J. Dev. Behav. Pediatr.* **2017**, *38*, 135–150. [CrossRef] [PubMed]
7. Gregory, C.A.; Coleman-Jensen, A. *Food Insecurity, Chronic Disease, and Health Among Working-Age Adults*; US Department of Agriculture, Economic Research Service: Washington, DC, USA, 2017.
8. Gundersen, C.; Ziliak, J.P. Food insecurity and health outcomes. *Health Aff. (Millwood)* **2015**, *34*, 1830–1839. [CrossRef] [PubMed]
9. Laraia, B.A. Food insecurity and chronic disease. *Adv. Nutr.* **2013**, *4*, 203–212. [CrossRef] [PubMed]

10. Cook, J.T.; Black, M.; Chilton, M.; Cutts, D.; Ettinger de Cuba, S.; Heeren, T.C.; Rose-Jacobs, R.; Sandel, M.; Casey, P.H.; Coleman, S.; et al. Are food insecurity's health impacts underestimated in the U.S. population? Marginal food security also predicts adverse health outcomes in young U.S. children and mothers. *Adv. Nutr.* **2013**, *4*, 51–61. [CrossRef] [PubMed]
11. Cook, J.T.; Frank, D.A.; Berkowitz, C.; Black, M.M.; Casey, P.H.; Cutts, D.B.; Meyers, A.F.; Zaldivar, N.; Skalicky, A.; Levenson, S.; et al. Food insecurity is associated with adverse health outcomes among human infants and toddlers. *J. Nutr.* **2004**, *134*, 1432–1438. [CrossRef] [PubMed]
12. Cook, J.T.; Frank, D.A.; Levenson, S.M.; Neault, N.B.; Heeren, T.C.; Black, M.M.; Berkowitz, C.; Casey, P.H.; Meyers, A.F.; Cutts, D.B.; et al. Child food insecurity increases risks posed by household food insecurity to young children's health. *J. Nutr.* **2006**, *136*, 1073–1076. [CrossRef] [PubMed]
13. Mabli, J.; Ohls, J.; Dragoset, L.; Castner, L.; Santos, B. *Measuring the Effect of Supplemental Nutrition Assistance Program (SNAP) Participation on Food Security*; U.S. Department of Agriculture, Food and Nutrition Service: Alexandria, VA, USA, 2013.
14. Ratcliffe, C.; McKernan, S.M.; Zhang, S. How much does the supplemental nutrition assistance program reduce food insecurity? *Am. J. Agric. Econ.* **2011**, *93*, 1082–1098. [CrossRef] [PubMed]
15. Characteristics of USDA Supplemental Nutrition Assistance Program Households. Available online: www.fns.usda.gov/research-and-analysis (accessed on 29 March 2019).
16. Policy Basics: The Supplemental Nutrition Assistance Program (SNAP). Available online: https://www.cbpp.org/research/policy-basics-the-supplemental-nutrition-assistance-program-snap (accessed on 29 March 2019).
17. Nord, M.; Prell, M. *Food Security Improved Following the 2009 ARRA Increase in SNAP Benefits*; Economic Research Report # 116; U.S. Department of Agriculture: Washington, DC, USA, 2011.
18. Almond, D.; Hoynes, H.W.; Schanzenbach, D.W. Inside the war on poverty: The impact of food stamps on birth outcomes. *Rev. Econ. Stat.* **2011**, *93*, 387–403. [CrossRef]
19. Ettinger de Cuba, S.; Weiss, I.; Pasquariello, J.; Schiffmiller, A.; Frank, D.A.; Coleman, S.; Breen, A.; Cook, J.T. *The SNAP Vaccine: Boosting Children's Health*; Children's HealthWatch: Boston, MA, USA, 2012.
20. Kreider, B.; Pepper, J.V.; Gunderson, C.; Jolliffe, D. Identifying the effects of SNAP (food stamps) on child health outcomes when participation is endogenous and misreported. *J. Am. Stat. Assoc.* **2012**, *107*, 958–975. [CrossRef]
21. Mabli, J.; Worthington, J. Supplemental nutrition assistance program participation and child food security. *Pediatrics* **2014**, *133*, 610–619. [CrossRef] [PubMed]
22. Mabli, J.; Ohls, J. Supplemental nutrition assistance program participation is associated with an increase in household food security in a national evaluation. *J. Nutr.* **2015**, *145*, 344–351. [CrossRef] [PubMed]
23. Bitler, M.; Hoynes, H. Immigrants, welfare reform and the U.S. safety net. *NBER Working Pap. Ser.* **2011**. [CrossRef]
24. Capps, R.; Fix, M.; Ost, J.; Reardon-Anderson, J.; Passel, J.S. *The Health and Well-Being of Young Children of Immigrants*; The Urban Institute: Washington, DC, USA, 2005.
25. Van Hook, J.; Balistreri, K.S. Ineligible parents, eligible children: Food stamps receipt, allotments, and food insecurity among children of immigrants. *Soc. Sci. Res.* **2006**, *35*, 228–251. [CrossRef]
26. Capps, R.; Chishti, M.; Gelatt, J.; Bolter, J.; Ruiz Soto, A.G. *Revving Up the Deportation Machinery: Enforcement under Trump and the Pushback*; Migration Policy Institute: Washington, DC, USA, 2018.
27. López, G.; Bialik, K.; Radford, J. Key Findings about U.S Immigrants. Available online: http://www.pewresearch.org/fact-tank/2018/11/30/key-findings-about-u-s-immigrants/ (accessed on 3 March 2019).
28. Evich, H.M. Immigrants, Fearing Trump Crackdown, Drop out of Nutrition Programs. *Politico*, 3 September 2018. Available online: https://www.politico.com/story/2018/09/03/immigrants-nutrition-food-trump-crackdown-806292 (accessed on 3 March 2019).
29. Dewey, C. Immigrants are Going Hungry so Trump Won't Deport Them. *The Washington Post*, 16 March 2017. Available online: https://www.washingtonpost.com/news/wonk/wp/2017/03/16/immigrants-are-now-canceling-their-food-stamps-for-fear-that-trump-will-deport-them/?utm_term=.99340832c097 (accessed on 25 February 2019).
30. Black, M.M.; Quigg, A.M.; Cook, J.T.; Casey, P.H.; Cutts, D.B.; Chilton, M.; Meyers, A.; Ettinger de Cuba, S.; Heeren, T.; Coleman, S.; et al. WIC participation and attenuation of stress-related child health risks of household food insecurity and caregiver depressive symptoms. *Arch. Pediatr. Adolesc. Med.* **2012**, *166*, 444–451. [CrossRef] [PubMed]

31. Cutts, D.B.; Meyers, A.F.; Black, M.M.; Casey, P.H.; Chilton, M.; Cook, J.T.; Geppert, J.; Ettinger de Cuba, S.; Heeren, T.; Coleman, S. US housing insecurity and the health of very young children. *Am. J. Public Health* **2011**, *101*, 1508–1514. [CrossRef] [PubMed]
32. Ettinger de Cuba, S.; Chilton, M.; Bovell-Ammon, A.; Knowles, M.; Coleman, S.; Black, M.M.; Cook, J.T.; Cutts, D.B.; Casey, P.H.; Heeren, T.C.; Frank, D.A. Loss of SNAP is associated with food insecurity and poor health in working families with young children. *Health Aff. (Millwood)* **2019**, Forthcoming.
33. Bonn, T. Trump's Immigration rhetoric has 'chilling effect' on families, says children's advocacy group director. *The Hill*, 20 December 2018. Available online: https://thehill.com/hilltv/rising/422371-childrens-advocacy-group-director-says-trumps-immigration-rhetoric-has-chilling (accessed on 3 March 2019).
34. Swetlitz, I. Immigrants, Fearing Trump's Deportation Policies, Avoid Doctor Visits. *Stat*, 24 February 2017. Available online: https://www.statnews.com/2017/02/24/immigrants-doctors-medical-care/ (accessed on 3 March 2019).
35. Green, E. First, They Excluded the Irish. *The Atlantic*, February 2017. Available online: https://www.theatlantic.com/politics/archive/2017/02/trump-poor-immigrants-public-charge/515397/ (accessed on 3 March 2019).
36. Hauslohner, A.; Ross, J. Trump administration circulates more draft immigration restrictions, focusing on protecting U.S jobs. *The Washington Post*, 31 January 2017. Available online: https://www.washingtonpost.com/world/national-security/trump-administration-circulates-more-draft-immigration-restrictions-focusing-on-protecting-us-jobs/2017/01/31/38529236-e741-11e6-80c2-30e57e57e05d_story.html?utm_term=.7359cd55708d (accessed on 3 March 2019).
37. Cook, J.T.; Poblacion, A. *Estimating the Health-Related Costs of Food Insecurity and Hunger*; Bread for the World Institute: Washington, DC, USA, 2016.
38. Berkowitz, S.A.; Basu, S.; Meigs, J.B.; Seligman, H. Food Insecurity and Health Care Expenditures in the United States, 2011–2013. *Health Serv. Res.* **2017**, *53*, 1600–1620. [CrossRef] [PubMed]
39. Yoshikawa, H.; Chaudry, A.; García, S.R.; Koball, H.; Francis, T. *Approaches to Protect Children's Access to Health and Human Services in an Era of Harsh Immigration Policy*; New York University: New York City, NY, USA, 2019.

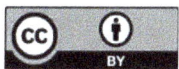

© 2019 by the authors. Licensee MDPI, Basel, Switzerland. This article is an open access article distributed under the terms and conditions of the Creative Commons Attribution (CC BY) license (http://creativecommons.org/licenses/by/4.0/).

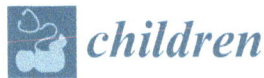

Article

Child Morbidity and Disease Burden in Refugee Camps in Mainland Greece

Asterios Kampouras [1,*], Georgios Tzikos [2], Eustathios Partsanakis [3], Konstantinos Roukas [4], Stefanos Tsiamitros [3], Dimitrios Deligeorgakis [3], Elisavet Chorafa [5], Maria Schoina [6] and Elias Iosifidis [7]

1. Pediatric Department, 424 General Military Hospital, Thessaloniki 56429, Greece
2. Surgery Department, 424 General Military Hospital, Thessaloniki 56429, Greece; giorgos-t@hotmail.com
3. Medical Service, Hellenic Army, Thessaloniki 56429, Greece; epartsa@gmail.com (E.P.); stevetsam@gmail.com (S.T.); d.deligeorgakis@gmail.com (D.D.)
4. Internal Medicine Department, 424 General Military Hospital, Thessaloniki 56429, Greece; rooky17@gmail.com
5. School of Medicine, Aristotle University of Thessaloniki, Thessaloniki 54124, Greece; elsachorafa@hotmail.gr
6. Nephrology Department, Hippokration General Hospital, Aristotle University of Thessaloniki, Thessaloniki 54642, Greece; maninaschoina@gmail.com
7. Infection Control Committee, Hippokration General Hospital, Infectious Diseases Unit, 3rd Department of Pediatrics, Aristotle University of Thessaloniki, Thessaloniki 54642, Greece; iosifidish@gmail.com
* Correspondence: asterioskampouras@gmail.com; Tel.: +30-23-1038-1000

Received: 11 February 2019; Accepted: 8 March 2019; Published: 17 March 2019

Abstract: The crisis conflicts in Syria have forced a lot of people to relocate and live in mainland Greece, where they are hosted in refugee camps. In the present study, our aim was to assess child morbidity and overall disease burden in two camps in northern Greece during a six-month winter period. A primary health care office was founded in each camp. Refugees of all ages with health problems were examined daily by specialty doctors. Cases were classified into two categories: Infectious or non-infectious. In total, 2631 patients were examined during this period (out of the 3760 refugees hosted). Of these patients, 9.8% were infants, 12.7% were toddlers, and 13.4% were children. Most of the visits for children aged less than 12 years old were due to infectious diseases (80.8%). The most common sites of communicable diseases among children were the respiratory tract (66.8%), the skin (23.2%), and the urinary (3.2%) and gastrointestinal tracts (6.2%). Non-communicable diseases were mostly due to gastrointestinal (20.2%), respiratory (18.2%), surgical (13.1%), and allergic (10.3%) disorders. Infants, toddlers, and children suffered more frequently from respiratory infections, while in adolescents and adults, non-infectious diseases were more common. Toddlers and children were more likely to fall ill in comparison to infants. Conclusions: During the winter period, infectious diseases, especially of the respiratory tract, are the main reason for care seeking among refugees in Greek camps, with toddlers suffering more than other age groups. The overall mortality and referral percentage were low, indicating that adequate primary care is provided in this newly established refugee hosting model.

Keywords: child morbidity; disease burden; refugee crisis

1. Introduction

The ongoing crisis with the intense conflicts in Syria and neighboring countries has forced more than 6 million people to abandon their home countries, seeking a safer place to relocate to [1]. The deteriorating situation in Syria accounts for the increased amount of refugees, whose primary destinations are countries in central and northern Europe, which they have tried to reach by following the eastern Mediterranean route through Turkey and Greece [1,2]. However, the closure of the Greek-Former Yugoslav Republic of Macedonia (FYROM) border on February 2016 has caused the popular "Balkan route" to shut down. Refugees and migrants, for whom Greece was mainly a transitional location, had their dream interrupted [3]. Adding to that, the implementation of the EU-Turkey agreement on March 2016 drastically limited the arrival of more refugees to Greece, who instead will likely try to reach Europe through irregular ways, risking their lives [2–4]. As a result, more than 62,000 refugees are currently stranded in Greece, with no prospect of moving to any northern countries [5].

Moreover, refugee camps (or "hotspots"), originally aimed for short-term stays, had to be turned into long-term shelters, and since they were not designed to host such large amounts of refugees, they became overcrowded. Therefore, new challenges have arisen as the facilities are not adequate, thus the living conditions are considered inappropriate. Another important issue that has come up is that these camps may host a considerable number of unaccompanied minors, especially children with an unknown vaccination status, suffering from the war and the uncertainty of the journey to a new place to resettle. Consequently, both their physical and mental health have been disturbed [6]. These facts raise questions about the burden of disease and the prevalence of vaccine-preventable diseases. Lately, there has been increased interest and a need for evidence-based reports on migrant health and its impact on the national health systems of European countries [7,8], along with a lack of adequate data on the health condition of the current refugee wave.

Therefore, the aim of the present study was to: (a) assess the burden of disease in two refugee camps in mainland northern Greece during an autumn-winter period, and (b) compare the burden of disease between different age groups, also checking child morbidity.

2. Methods

Our study was conducted in two refugee camps in northern Greece during the autumn-winter period from October 2016 to March 2017. These camps hosted about 250 refugees each, who had mostly travelled from Afghanistan and Syria. Of these refugees, about 280 were adults, and about 220 were under 18 years old. Refugees arrive at these camps a few days after entering the country, usually by sea. Upon entrance they are vaccinated, according to the National Immunization Schedule, and after asylum is granted to them they are relocated to camps in mainland Greece, in order to avoid congestion at entrance points. In refugee camps in mainland Greece, refugees stay for an average period of 1.5 months until they find housing in one of Greece's cities. Most of the children who arrive are accompanied by family members. The status of previous vaccination was undefined in most cases. A primary health care office was founded in every camp and was ran under the supervision of the medical service of the Hellenic Army. Refugees with health problems were examined on a daily basis by specialty doctors and were referred to tertiary or university hospitals when further care was needed. In cases of emergency, patients were transferred to hospitals with the assistance of ambulances from the National Emergency Aid Center. Communicable diseases were categorized into four groups according to the site of the infection, which included respiratory, urinary, gastrointestinal, and skin infections. In cases of febrile illness, C-Reactive Protein (CRP) values were measured on site. Regarding non-communicable diseases, patients were also classified in categories according to the system that was affected (cardiovascular, surgical, obstetric, gastrointestinal, respiratory, allergic, orthopedic, hematological, endocrinological, or others). A database of refugees providing medical care was created with the following fields: Age, gender, reason for seeking medical advice, underlying condition, medical diagnosis, CRP, and referrals. Each patient was recorded once every time they sought medical advice in order to avoid duplicate recorded data. All patients were informed about the study and provided informed written consent. All procedures performed in this study involving human participants were in accordance with the ethical standards of the institutional or national research committee and with the 1964 Helsinki declaration and its later amendments or comparable ethical standards.

Statistical Analysis

Statistical analysis was conducted with the help of the IBM SPSS statistics software (24th edition). Baseline characteristics were summarized using appropriate descriptive statistics. The statistical significance was set to 0.05. The chi-square test was used to efficiently determine whether there was any association between the presence of infection or any other pathological condition status and different age groups, due to the fact that the variables were categorical. Finally, logistic regression was used to assess if there were any significant associations between the type of infection or pathological condition and different age groups.

3. Results

3.1. Demographics

During the period from October 2016 to March 2017, approximately 3760 refugees found shelter in the two camps of our study, with 1654 of them being children (approximately 334 were infants (which accounts for 8% of whole population), 648 were toddlers (17%), and 672 were children (18%) 6–12 years old). In total, 2631 patients were examined at the primary care office. About 9.8% of them were infants, whereas 12.7% were toddlers. Children aged 6–12 years old accounted for 13.4% of office visits, whereas adolescents (12–18 years old) accounted for 7.9%. The age group of adults who were examined consisted of 1453 patients (55.2%). (Table 1) Regarding their gender, 48.2% of the refugees seeking medical care were male and 51.8% were female.

Table 1. Demographic Data.

Age Group	N (%)
Infants	258 (9.8)
Toddlers	333 (12.7)
Children	353 (13.4)
Adolescents	209 (7.9)
Adults	1453 (55.2)
Total	2631 (100)

3.2. Care Seeking or Reason for Care Seeking

The most common reason for care seeking among the entire population was due to an infectious disease (58.4%). Regarding the rest of cases for care seeking, 41.6% were for non-communicable or non-infectious diseases. Regarding infectious diseases, the most common site of infection was the respiratory tract (64.2%), followed by the skin and soft tissue (21.9%), the urinary tract (6.7%), and the gastrointestinal tract (6.3%) (Figure 1). There were also 14 refugees (0.9%) with more than one infection.

For non-infectious conditions, cardiovascular (19.5%), surgical (6.0%), obstetrics-gynecological (8.5%), gastrointestinal (12.5%), respiratory (3.2%), allergic (4.3%), orthopedic (14.7%), hematological (2.6%), and endocrinological (1.9%) disorders were observed. About 26.2% of patients with non-infectious diseases who were seeking care were examined by doctors for different reasons (e.g., consultation, diet guidance), and 0.9% of them suffered from more than one condition (Figure 2).

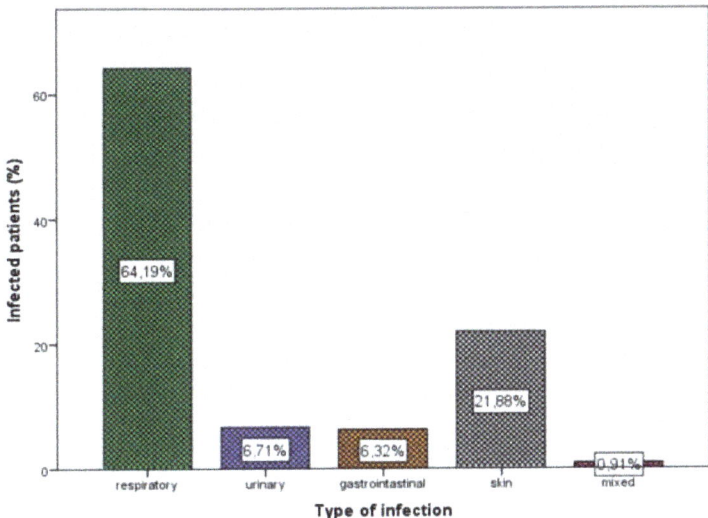

Figure 1. Type and percentage of infection in the whole population.

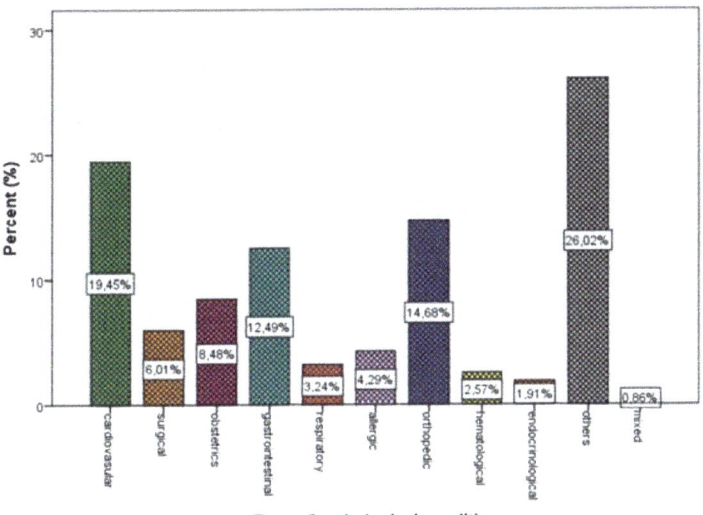

Figure 2. Percentage of system affected in non-infectious diseases for the whole population.

3.3. Child Morbidity

Types of infections among children are shown in Figure 3.

Respiratory track infection was the most common disease in the age groups of infants (48.8%), toddlers (54.4%), and children (58.9%) (Table 2). On the other hand, in the age groups of adolescents (49.8%) and adults (55.3%), the most frequent reason for medical advice or care seeking was a non-infectious or non-communicable condition or disease.

It is worth mentioning that toddlers were 1.564 times ($p = 0.027$) more likely to get ill comparing to infants (Table 2).

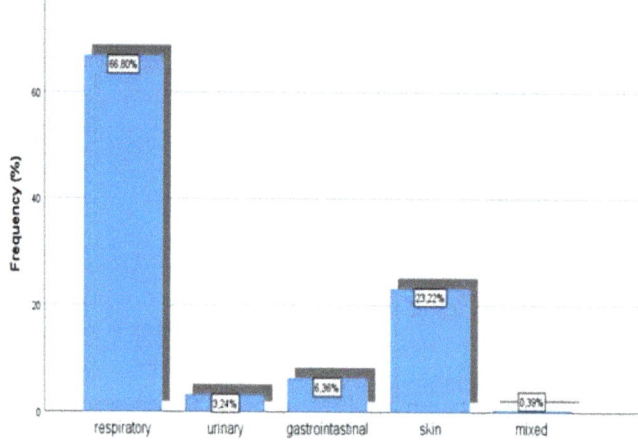

Figure 3. Types of infections among infants, toddlers, and children.

Table 2. Relative risk of suffering from an infectious disease among age groups.

	p	RR	95% C.I.	
			Lower	Upper
Toddlers vs. Infants_	0.027	1,564	1,053	2,325
Children vs. Infants	0.069	1,428	973	2,097

However, statistical analysis revealed that there was no association between gender and morbidity ($p = 0.422$). (RR: Relative Risk, C.I.: Confidence Interval)

Odds ratio and confidence intervals for overall morbidity in comparison to infants are shown on Figure 4. Toddlers were about 1.564 times more likely to get sick than infants, whereas children were 1.4 times more likely to get sick.

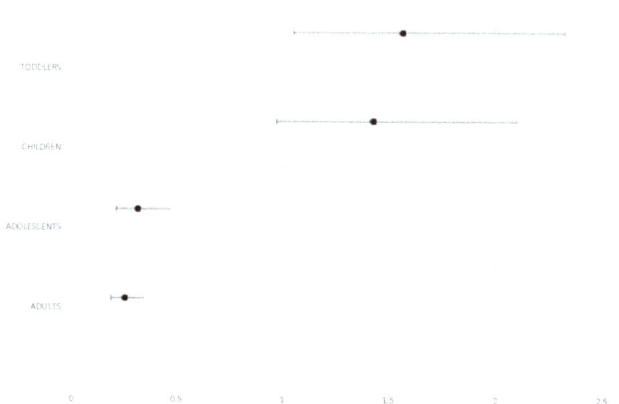

Figure 4. Odds ratio and CI for overall morbidity in comparison to the age group of infants.

Lastly, only 1.4% of the patients who were examined were taken to hospital for further examination and treatment.

4. Discussion

The main finding of our study is that during a 6-month winter period, most of the children's visits to the doctor's office in refugee camps were due to infectious diseases (66,8%). Respiratory tract infections accounted for the majority of communicable diseases, with toddlers being more likely to suffer from one in comparison to the other age groups. Despite this relatively high morbidity due to infectious diseases, the percentage of referrals to tertiary hospitals was significantly low, and no serious cases of vaccine-preventable disease outbreaks and mortality were noted.

This finding comes in accordance with the results of other studies conducted over the last decade, in which infectious diseases are mentioned as the main health problem between asylum seekers [8,9]. In a very recent study that took place in Greece, members of Syrian American Medical Society Global Response (SAMS—GR), who provided medical services in four refugee camps in northern Greece, examined about 7500 people of all ages over a three-month summer period (June 2016–August 2016), most of whom were also adults [10]. Female patients (51.8%) outnumbered the male ones (48.2%). In the aforementioned study, respiratory and gastrointestinal infections were the main reason for care seeking among refugees in Northern Greece.

Analyzing our infection data bank, diseases of respiratory tract were the most common among other conditions. Of all patients, 37.5% were diagnosed with a respiratory infection, while 12.8% had skin infections. Urinary and gastrointestinal infections accounted for only 3.9% and 3.7% of all infectious diseases, respectively, which indicates that overall hygiene conditions in the camps were of a relatively good level. Only 14 patients (0.5%) were diagnosed with more than one infection. Multimorbidity was also negatively associated with immigrants and refugees in another study [11]. Previous studies which took place in Greece and Brussels also reported that respiratory symptoms were the most common finding among the patients [9–12]. The resettlement of asylum seekers to a different environment and the exposure to other respiratory viruses may explain this fact [13]. Similar findings (especially respiratory, digestive, and skin conditions among newly arrived refugees) were also reported in other studies [9–12]. A possible explanation for the prevalence of these diseases might be the poor state of migrants' health and the questionable hygienic conditions during their travel [8,12,14]. Overcrowded camps and poor living conditions may have made migrants more vulnerable to communicable illnesses as well, especially from the respiratory and gastrointestinal system [8–15]. In their study, Bloch-Infanger et al. claim that the percentage of the migrant population seeking for medical care has increased among young people during the last decade [8]. Furthermore, these patients were most frequently referred and hospitalized [8]. Despite the fact that communicable diseases were the most common reason for care seeking in the population of our study, overall referrals to tertiary hospitals were very few. This may be an indicator of adequate first level medical care and easy access to the doctor's office. Appropriate access to medical care regardless of the legal status of each country is vital in order to improve health status and enhance the prevention of contagious diseases [16].

Regarding non-infectious conditions (41.62%), these were classified in eleven categories based on system affected: cardiovascular (19.45%), surgical (6.01%), obstetrics-gynecological (8.48%), gastrointestinal (12.49%), respiratory (3.2%), allergic (4.29%), orthopedic (14.68%), hematological (2.57%), and endocrinological (1.91%). Approximately 26.02% of patients were examined by doctors for different reasons and 0.86% had more than one pathological issue. Some studies indicate that chronic diseases and psychiatric conditions are the most important health problems among migrants and refugees hosted in camps [17,18]. In our study, neither chronic disorders, such as Hepatitis A, B, or C infections and tuberculosis, nor mental issues, such as depression, were observed. Lastly, no patients with dental problems sought medical care, in contrast to van Berlaer et al., who reported 10% of refugees had dental issues and visited the doctor's office [9], and a study which took place at P. and A. Kyriakou Children's Hospital, a tertiary pediatric hospital in Athens, Greece, which showed that between immigrant children who were examined clinically at the hospital, dental abnormalities (21%) were the most frequent medical problem identified. In our study, other disorders, such as respiratory and dermatological infections, genitourinary, cardiological, and surgical matters requiring further intervention, existed in 7.3% of this research population. [19]. We have to clarify that long-term conditions (including vector-borne and blood-borne infections, such as malaria, leishmaniasis, and *Helicobacter Pylori*) may have been underrepresented or under-diagnosed, as health care providers focused on identifying acute conditions.

In our study, we also compared the disease burden among different age groups. This comparison revealed that respiratory infections are the most common disease in the age groups of infants (48.8%), toddlers (54.4%), and children (58.9%), whereas in the age groups of adolescents (49.8%) and adults (55.3%), the most frequent disorder is non-infectious. Pavli et al. also reported that refugee children are prone to respiratory and gastrointestinal issues, as well as skin conditions [12]. In our study, we examined the relative chance for infection between age groups and we found out that toddlers were 1.564 times ($p = 0.027$) and children were 1.428 times ($p = 0.069$) more likely to suffer from communicable diseases compared to infants (Figure 4). This comes in accordance with other studies as well. For instance, van Berlaer et al. reported that almost two-thirds of children younger than 5 years of age suffered from diseases [9]. Lastly, our study shows that there is no association whatsoever between gender and likelihood of someone getting sick. Even though some studies report female immigrants being more vulnerable to health disorders, in our study no such association was noted [12].

To our knowledge, this is the first study examining disease burden and child morbidity in Greek refugee camps during a 6-month winter period. Refugee camps in mainland Greece were established in a very short period of time with few resources, mainly as temporary dwellings that were meant to accommodate people for short-term stays only. However, the closure of the "Balkan route" and the EU-Turkey agreement has lead Greek refugee camps to become overcrowded long-term shelters overnight. This new refugee sheltering model, along with the fact that conflicts in Syria are still in progress, has prompted the need to have its functionality and effectiveness assessed, especially in terms of medical care and morbidity. Thus, our study fills a gap in the existing literature shedding light on the overall disease burden during the winter period and examining how child groups shoulder this burden.

A number of limitations exist. Even though we excluded from our database double reports for the same patient and condition, there were patients visiting the primary care office two or three times, thus not allowing for the overall risk to be calculated. Additionally, we focused on the group of children less than 12 years old and excluded adolescents (who in terms of infectious diseases demonstrate more common morbidity to adults) from our analysis. A study that could compare refugee morbidity to that of the local population would provide better understanding of the overall disease burden and guide possible prevention interventions.

In conclusion, communicable diseases are the most common cause for care seeking among refugees in camps in mainland Greece during a winter period, with children and especially toddlers suffering more often from respiratory tract illnesses than other age groups. This urgently-established refugee hosting model in Greece seems to be working effectively in terms of primary medical care and hygiene levels.

Author Contributions: Conceptualization, A.K.; data curation, G.T., E.P., D.D., E.C., and M.S.; formal analysis, G.T. and E.I.; investigation, E.P.; methodology, A.K.; project administration, A.K.; supervision, A.K.; validation, M.S. and E.I.; writing—original draft, E.P., K.R., S.T., and D.D.; writing—review and editing, A.K. and E.I.

Conflicts of Interest: The authors declare no conflict of interest.

References

1. United Nations High Commissioner for Refugees. Desperate Journeys. Available online: http://www.unhcr.org/news/updates/2017/2/58b449f54/desperate-journeys-refugees-migrants-entering-crossing-europe-via-mediterranean.html (accessed on 11 February 2019).
2. Syria: Crisis Update—28 November 2016. Available online: http://www.msf.org/en/articles/syria-crisis-update-28-november-2016 (accessed on 11 February 2019).
3. World Health Organization. Europe-Migration and Health. Available online: http://www.euro.who.int/en/health-topics/health-determinants/migration-and-health/news/news/2017/03/a-journey-interrupted-the-changing-health-needs-of-refugees-and-migrants-stranded-in-greece (accessed on 11 February 2019).
4. European Commission-Fact Sheet. EU-Turkey Statement: Questions and Answers. Available online: http://europa.eu/rapid/press-releaseMEMO-16-963en.html (accessed on 11 February 2019).
5. United Nations High Commissioner for Refugees. Greece FactSheet-May 2017. Available online: https://data2.unhcr.org/en/documents/details/58264 (accessed on 11 February 2019).
6. Save the Children-Invisible Wounds. Available online: http://www.savethechildren.org.uk/sites/default/files/images/InvissibleWounds.pdf (accessed on 11 February 2019).
7. Khan, M.S.; Osei-Kofi, A.; Omar, A.; Kirkbride, H.; Kessel, A.; Abbara, A.; Heymann, D.; Zumla, A.; Dar, O. Pathogens, prejudice, and politics: The role of the global health community in the European refugee crisis. *Lancet Infect. Dis.* **2016**, *16*, e173–e177. [CrossRef]
8. Bloch-Infanger, C.; Battig, V.; Kremo, J.; Widmer, A.F.; Egli, A.; Bingisser, R.; Battegay, M.; Erb, S. Increasing prevalence of infectious diseases in asylum seekers at a tertiary care hospital in Switzerland. *PLoS ONE* **2017**, *12*, e0179537. [CrossRef] [PubMed]
9. Van Berlaer, G.; Bohle Carbonell, F.; Manantsoa, S.; de Bethune, X.; Buyl, R.; Debacker, M.; Hubloue, I. A refugee camp in the centre of Europe: Clinical characteristics of asylum seekers arriving in Brussels. *BMJ Open* **2016**, *6*, e013963. [CrossRef] [PubMed]
10. Abbara, A.; Jarman, K.; Isreb, M.; Gunst, M.; Sahloul, Z.M. Models similar to the Refugees' Health Unit exist in northern Greece. *Lancet* **2016**, *388*, 2352. [CrossRef]
11. Diaz, E.; Poblador-Pou, B.; Gimeno-Feliu, L.-A.; Calderón-Larrañaga, A.; Kumar, B.N.; Prados-Torres, A. Multimorbidity and Its Patterns according to Immigrant Origin. A Nationwide Register-Based Study in Norway. *PLoS ONE* **2015**, *10*, e0145233. [CrossRef] [PubMed]
12. Pavli, A.; Maltezou, H. Health problems of newly arrived migrants and refugees in Europe. *J. Travel Med.* **2017**, *24*. [CrossRef] [PubMed]
13. Stich, A. Coming in to the cold – Access to health care is urgently needed for Syrian refugees. *Travel Med. Infect. Dis.* **2015**, *13*, 445–446. [CrossRef] [PubMed]
14. Soares, A.A.; Tzafalias, M. Europe gears up to attend to refugees' health. *Bull. World Health Org.* **2015**, *93*, 822–823. [PubMed]
15. Daynes, L. The health impacts of the refugee crisis: A medical charity perspective. *Clin. Med.* **2016**, *16*, 437–440. [CrossRef] [PubMed]
16. Castelli, F.; Sulis, G. Migration and infectious diseases—Clinical microbiology and infection. *Off. Publ. Eur. Soc. Clin. Microbiol. Infect. Dis.* **2017**, *23*, 283–289. [CrossRef] [PubMed]
17. Dookeran, N.M.; Battaglia, T.; Cochran, J.; Geltman, P.L. Chronic disease and its risk factors among refugees and asylees in Massachusetts, 2001–2005. *Prev. Chronic Dis.* **2010**, *7*, A51.
18. Fazel, M.; Wheeler, J.; Danesh, J. Prevalence of serious mental disorder in 7000 refugees resettled in western countries: A systematic review. *Lancet* **2005**, *365*, 1309–1314. [CrossRef]
19. Pavlopoulou, I.D.; Tanaka, M.; Dikalioti, S.; Samoli, E.; Nisianakis, P.; Boleti, O.D.; Tsoumakas, K. Clinical and laboratory evaluation of new immigrant and refugee children arriving in Greece. *BMC Pediatr.* **2017**, *17*, 132. [CrossRef] [PubMed]

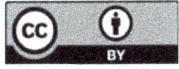

© 2019 by the authors. Licensee MDPI, Basel, Switzerland. This article is an open access article distributed under the terms and conditions of the Creative Commons Attribution (CC BY) license (http://creativecommons.org/licenses/by/4.0/).

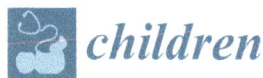

Article

Addressing Marginality and Exclusion: The Resettlement Experiences of War-Affected Young People in Quebec, Canada

Andie (Saša) Buccitelli [1],* and Myriam Denov [2],*

1. Social Service Program, Dawson College, Montreal, QC H3Z 1A4, Canada
2. School of Social Work, McGill University, Montreal, QC H3A 2A7, Canada
* Correspondence: abuccitelli@dawsoncollege.qc.ca (A.S.B.); myriam.denov@mcgill.ca (M.D.)

Received: 18 December 2018; Accepted: 27 January 2019; Published: 30 January 2019

Abstract: Accessing meaningful forms of support can be an onerous experience for young people resettling from war-affected contexts. In addition to facing linguistic and financial barriers in this process, these young people negotiate care systems that are often structurally and culturally insensitive to their unique needs, values, beliefs, and intersectional experiences of oppression. Drawing on interviews with 22 young people from war-affected areas living in Quebec, Canada, this paper critically examines how dominant cultural norms and social relations in Quebec's health, social and educational services network shape their experiences in seeking care, healing and belonging. Alternative care systems and approaches, as proposed by the participants, are then explored. The findings emphasize the need for spaces and care services where war-affected young people's identities and lived realities are validated and represented.

Keywords: war; migration; resettlement; refugee; youth; exclusion; cultural norms; Quebec; Canada

---

1. Introduction

Wars continue to alter the lives of children, young people, and families around the world with devastating social, economic, political and psychological effects. More than 600 million, or one in four, of the world's youth, live in areas affected by armed conflict and insecurity [1]. Within these wartime contexts, children and young people are killed, exploited, abused, injured, orphaned, separated from family and/or recruited into armed groups (for the purpose of this study, "child" is defined as any person under the age of 18 years, in accordance with the United Nations *Convention on the Rights of the Child* (UNCRC), while "young person" is defined as anyone between 15 and 30 years of age).

Countries like Canada are indirectly, yet intimately touched by war. Each year, thousands of children enter Canada, fleeing war zones [2]. Refugees admitted to Canada represent approximately 10% of the roughly 285,000 new permanent residents in the country every year [3]. In 2016, the United Nations High Commissioner for Refugees (UNHCR) lauded Canada's resettlement of 46,700 refugees, a record high in refugees admitted since the implementation of the 1976 Immigration Act [4]. This represents a 133% increase compared to the previous year. Additionally, nearly half (47%) of refugees admitted to Canada in 2016 were children [5]. In the year of 2017, the Government of Canada reported a total of 50,380 asylum claimants (processed across the country (it is worth noting the shift in language, using 'asylum claims' instead of the terms 'refugee claim'/ 'refugee claimant' as used in the Immigration and Refugee Protection Act). Based on recent figures reported by Immigration, Refugees and Citizenship Canada (IRCC), as of 29 January 2017, Canada resettled a total of 40,081 Syrian refugees [5]. This is due in part to Canada's humanitarian transfer of Syrian refugees with UNHCR's support, as part of the Canadian government's explicit commitment to resettle refugees with a "renewed focus on reuniting families" [5]. The government has also emphasized the importance of combined efforts with civil society and service providers to support refugees' resettlement and integration [4].

Resettlement from a war-affected context is both complex and multifaceted. Young people displaced from war zones witness or directly experience severe and unimaginable violence and upheaval. For those who make their way to Canada, war-related mental health distress may occur alongside poverty, discrimination, isolation, language barriers and difficulties in school [6,7]. Studies on young people with refugee backgrounds in Australia point to similar resettlement realities [8–17]. With growing numbers of asylum claimants and their families receiving permanent residency—and becoming interwoven in the Canadian social fabric—it is critical that psychosocial programs and interventions address their needs, as individuals, families and communities. Moreover, there is a greater need for culturally responsive practice with children and families from war-affected and refugee backgrounds that accounts for the diversity and heterogeneity of their needs and experiences.

The province of Quebec has a unique independence with regard to immigration policies since the signing of the Canada-Quebec accord in 1994. This accord allows the province to develop its own criteria for selecting immigrants and refugees from abroad. However, under this accord, Canada remains in charge of the selection and processing of asylum seekers. The accord was negotiated in order to ensure the promotion of the French language and the uniqueness of Quebec's cultural identity. It also set Quebec apart from Canada by its use of an intercultural model rather than a multicultural model within the policy [18].

There is an emerging literature on the experiences of young people with refugee backgrounds and from war-affected areas in multiple contexts around the world [8–17], including Canada [7,19–23]. However, the lived realities, resettlement experiences and service provision needs of this population of children and young people deserve greater attention and ensuing action. In particular, how do young people from war-affected countries living in Quebec negotiate resettlement? How and where do these young people seek support? How do young people experience support in more formal spaces, including those integrated as part of Quebec's health, social services, and education systems? Answering these questions is key to informing and improving resettlement programs and services.

In exploring these experiences, this paper adopts the theoretical framework of intersectionality. Intersectionality posits that people's realities are shaped by the interaction of multiple forms of oppression (e.g., racism, sexism, ableism and classism), creating entirely new and unique experiences of marginalization [24–26]. Moreover, intersectionality supports an understanding of individuals' identities and experiences of oppression as fluid and mutable [27]. This is integral when exploring the complexities of individuals' social locations in light of migration and the shifting experience of oppression when accessing different spaces. This perspective is also useful in considering how historical processes of oppression impact the spaces young people navigate in the present (e.g., colonialism) [27]. In adopting an intersectional framework, this paper will critically explore how different forms of structural oppression, including insecurity, linguistic discrimination, racism, status and assimilation, shape war-affected young people's wellbeing and experiences in accessing support in different settings. Specifically, the paper aims to consider how dominant cultural paradigms and social relations in different systems and spaces affect young people's experiences of healing, support and exclusion.

2. Methodology

To examine the resettlement experiences of young people affected by war living in Quebec, in-depth interviews were conducted with 22 young people (11 male and 11 female) living in Montreal and St-Hyacinthe, a small-sized city located approximately 60 km east of Montreal (ethical approval number: #116-0912). These two contexts were chosen as they provide a glimpse into an urban setting and a more rural, or semi-rural, setting. Moreover, both contexts had relatively large numbers of war-affected young people with refugee backgrounds. The young people were recruited through the assistance of local settlement workers, and social workers. In addition, after interviewing several young people, we relied on snowball sampling to reach other potential participants. Participants were between the ages of 15 and 30 at the time of the interview/focus group and had been living in Canada from 6 months to 12 years. Their countries of origin included Colombia, Democratic Republic of Congo, Nepal, Rwanda, Sierra Leone, Sri Lanka, Togo and Zimbabwe and were conducted over a 10-month period, beginning in January 2013. Interviews were carried out in French, English or Spanish, depending upon participants' language preference. All interviews were audio-recorded with permission and subsequently transcribed.

The interviews were conducted by the second author, alongside a team of researchers involved in the project. Interviews took place at community centres or in the office of the researchers and lasted between one and two hours. Given our desire to ensure participants' overall safety and security during the research process, we aimed to include young people who were in some way along the "healing" journey. In this sense, participants were perceived as "leaders" by local social workers and settlement workers, who assisted in participant outreach. Nonetheless, to ensure the safety and security of participants, support systems—in the form of ongoing support and interventions from the settlement workers and social workers who assisted with participant outreach—were put into place in the aftermath of interviews.

To ensure that the participants' perspectives were appropriately captured, six young people from war-affected areas (aged 17–25) acted as 'youth advisors' during the design phase of the research. These young people were all from Colombia, having sought refugee status in Canada as a result of the armed conflict, and had been living in Canada between 2 and 5 years. A preliminary group discussion, conducted by the second author, was held with these six young people that outlined the goals and objectives of the research and explained our desire to develop interview questions that would be relevant to pose to potential research participants. The youth advisors were then asked to participate in a group discussion that addressed the opportunities and challenges that they themselves had experienced when resettling in Canada. In addition, the youth advisors worked individually and collectively to devise sample interview questions that they felt would be important to ask young people from war-affected areas who recently resettled to Canada. Youth advisors also offered critical feedback on our overall research objectives and provided direction in terms of appropriate methodologies emphasizing the importance that the interviewers "be present and ready to listen." A key contribution of the youth advisors was their emphasis on the importance of talking about young people's wartime pasts, even if the project's focus was on the issue of resettlement. As one of the youth advisors explained:

> *It is important to know the circumstances of youth prior to their arrival in order to understand what they may need. Some youth may seem to be functioning and well on the outside but on the inside, they may have a lot of repressed emotions and feeling. Experiences lived [during war] are not forgotten and are therefore expressed in different ways.*

The interview protocol developed based on their feedback, explored young people's wartime lives and experiences in the context of their countries of origin, the impact and legacy of the war on their lives, both past and present, as well as the realities of flight and resettlement to Quebec, Canada. The interviews also explored participants' sources of support once in Canada, both informal and formal, including their experiences with social and health services, as well as their comfort levels in sharing their stories of war, migration, and resettlement (For the purpose of this paper, "formal" spaces include organisations and agencies that are integrated into the Quebec government's publicly-funded education, health and social service systems. Examples include hospitals, schools, public clinics, such as CLSCs (*centre local de services communautaires*), and youth protection agencies). In addition to interviews, two focus groups were conducted with the same young people who had been interviewed as part of the research project. These focus groups, conducted by the second author and two members of her research team, aimed to trace the diverse opportunities and challenges that they faced upon resettling.

Data were analysed using a grounded theory approach, whereby through inductive analysis of the data, researchers gained an understanding of the patterns that exist in the social world under study, that are firmly grounded in the experiences of the individuals acting in it [28]. To facilitate data analysis, a conceptual coding tree was created with the assistance of HyperResearch—a qualitative analysis software. Through ongoing data analysis, participants' experiences of both support and exclusion in formal and informal spaces emerged consistently in the young people's narratives. These themes are addressed in greater detail in the following section.

3. Navigating Resettlement: Experiences in "Formal" Spaces

People sometimes think you are so traumatized. But what makes it more traumatizing is the system. You understand what I'm saying? It's the system.

—David, participant.

The experiences of war, flight and resettlement have complex implications for people's social, emotional and mental state of being. Loneliness, isolation, feeling uprooted, uncertainty about the future and a generalised sense of insecurity and fear featured prominently in participants' stories. After settling in Quebec, these young people were also expected to negotiate their way around a variety of systems whose inherent norms are often experienced as unfamiliar and disconcerting. Quebec's education and health and social services systems play an important role in many of these young people's post-resettlement lives. In the province of Quebec most, if not all young people, must attend "*des classes d'acceuil*" ('welcome classes') and begin the process of "*francisation*" in order to learn French and become better "accustomed" to local values, culture and social relations [29,30].

Moreover, many young people coming from war-affected areas may be referred to health and social services in order to receive psychosocial support for mental-health issues related to war, displacement, flight and resettlement. However, research has shown that minorities and immigrant families in Canada significantly underutilize mental health services and instead seek support from community organizations [31,32]. What is the reason behind this?

In many ways, schools, clinics, such as CLSCs, and other public services offered provincially in Canada are meant to support opportunities for learning and healing. Therefore, referring, or requiring young people to access these spaces seems reasonable given their past experiences of violence and the challenges that come with negotiating a new sociocultural environment. Although these spaces may act as centres of healing, learning and support, to varying degrees, they may simultaneously be experienced as sites of racial oppression, and assimilation. Upon entering these spaces, participants often reported confronting norms, values and social relations that did not speak to their unique realities, invalidated their beliefs, and eclipsed their sense of identity.

3.1. Health and Social Services: Conflicting Paradigms of Wellness

Canada's health and social services systems have been said to be heavily rooted in a modernist, Western biomedical understanding of health and illness. The focus is largely on the individual and the use of scientific tools and methods to assess and address the manifestation of disease [33]. Treatment often involves "separating" a person deemed "mentally ill" from the rest of society, sometimes through the use of labels (i.e., diagnoses) and/or their literal segregation from others (e.g., institutionalization) [34].

In interacting with the health and social services system, many young people in our study were faced with this Western conceptualisation of mental health. A common presumption is that most of these young people have been traumatised by the experience of war, and stand to benefit from a psychosocial assessment, followed by some form of treatment (i.e., therapy and/or medication). Similar processes of medicalisation, whereby people from refugee backgrounds are treated as "traumatised" and "psychologically harmed", have been highlighted in studies exploring resettlement experiences in the Australian context [12,15]. Of course, these assumptions, along with their associated theories and diagnoses, stem from a particular sociocultural standpoint: The notion of "mental health" was developed in North America and Europe [34]. As this participant points out:

> *The system is very, very culturally biased. They are very ignorant. Because for them it's just—they have this theory [...]. People come here from a traumatized country and they became more traumatized now [...] Western theory—applying [...] Western theory, it doesn't apply to some of us.*
>
> (David)

Refugees affected by war are readily screened for Post-traumatic Stress Disorder (PTSD) [15,35,36]. Although it may be the case that many people affected by war exhibit PTSD-like symptoms, it does not necessarily mean that some form of psychosocial intervention is required or even desired [15]. In fact, many young people in the study did not feel any particular need to access mental health support and described how seeking "outside" support was a peculiar concept for them:

> *It's not like I come from a country where [formal mental health support] is in abundance, because it's not. They don't have sort of a psychosocial worker [...] Granted, the family unit from those countries is so strong that there is never ever a need to start going outside—seeking help outside.*
>
> (Andy)

> *I never saw a psychologist. I never saw a therapist. But I made it on my own mind, created my own survival until I made it.*
>
> (David)

> *I don't think someone can help me [...] Because I think what I feel is normal, no? What I mean by normal, it's like—what I feel is—it's supposed to happen.*
>
> (Jasmine)

Many participants did not view their emotional and mental state as something that required professional attention. Finding power in oneself to heal, and looking for support from family and loved ones, appeared to be more organic avenues for the participants. The last quote reflects a perspective of mental health that differs from the biomedical model: rather than viewing how a person feels after a traumatic experience as an issue, it is important to understand that these emotions are perfectly "normal" in light of the difficult circumstances they faced in the context of war and violence.

Other participants who had considered to use, or who had actually accessed formal mental health resources, shared their reflections about the impact and consequences of these services:

> *Okay, yes. So I arrive, I take another appointment and I cry and cry. Ah! Okay!, I said: "Finally, it's exhausting, this system! I'm never coming back... So, I told myself I should go see the psychologist—because me—maybe I had a preconceived idea of a psychologist who would tell me, who would listen to me and tell me: "Pa-pa-pa-pa! You are cured!" But then—after I asked myself: "What is illness?*
>
> (Naomi)

The following participant reflected upon whether a practitioner from Canada would be able to understand the context of the war in which she grew up:

> *And it's the institutions that are not ready, or are not specified. They are for everyone, for all people in the school. So...but now, if I go see a psychologist, I tell myself: "Are they really going to understand my situation? [...] Are they really ready to listen to me?"*
>
> (Anna)

These testimonies highlight how some formal spaces may be unprepared and ill-equipped to support these young people. Moreover, are these professionals engaging and critically considering the structural realities of racism and xenophobia and how they may impact upon their everyday practice, as well as the everyday lives of their clients? As this participant astutely states:

> [One] of my criticisms of social work is—I'm going to be straightforward, here. It's whites, educated […] How many people do you find in social work that are a minority? Maybe there are one or two. But how can you understand someone's culture if you have just studied it from you own perspective? […] Refugees come here, all they want is the support to have safety. But, no, they don't feel safe. Because the same people they're talking to are the same person who is in the system. Social workers here, one of the greatest biases they have is that they don't see it from the client's own view. They see it from their own theories.
>
> (David)

> [The] people who work in the system have to be trained to help cultural education. Because a lot of people that I have spoken to find these people are culturally ignorant. If you walk into a clinic and you cover your head, already they have some perception about you. If I walk into the clinic being black or whatever, I don't know, people have shared that with me.
>
> (David)

In this sense, in order for people to benefit from formal spaces, specifically those that are part of the nation's public system, it seems imperative that these spaces are experienced as secure, validating and relevant.

3.2. Education: Feelings of Exclusion and Marginalisation

The participants also encountered a variety of challenges in navigating educational institutions. Here too, many were faced with social relations, norms and rules that rendered them feeling "othered." This participant, who was forced to abandon his schooling for several years, due to the break out of the war in his country of origin, explained how he was discouraged from continuing with his high school education once settled in Canada:

> They told me that I would never go to university. And I said to them, "Why?" They said because you're 22 now and here you have to go through adult [high school] system. Well, I'll apply to [name of university] and tell them the reason why they should accept me. I wrote them a letter of intent on my own and sent it out to them. They accepted me.
>
> (David)

> I was traumatized about coming [to university]. Psychologically, I was traumatized […] once, I finished this paper. I handed in. [...] The professor called me and said […] to me "Are you the one who wrote this paper?" I said, "Yes, I studied the book and I wrote it." She said, "Because we have some doubts. Your colleagues are thinking somebody gave it to you." I said, "You see? Why would you question the fact that I wrote this? I've been here—this is my final year." I was so upset. I brought all the papers that I have written. She apologized. But I said, "You want to discourage me to drop out of University. Then you will put me in statistics as one African, or whatever immigrant population, this, this, this." And she apologized. And I was sitting like this, and she said, "I'm sorry." And I cried in her office.
>
> (David)

> The system equals racism. It includes [name of university], includes [name of university], includes the hospitals.
>
> (David)

> Because it's obvious that at school, they see us like an immigrant. It's there that I feel the difference between being an immigrant and you as a person, what you [experienced/lived through]. They see you as an immigrant, they always ask you the same question: "where do you come from?" always this. And they don't go much further than this. It doesn't go much further. Like … I don't know,

I have Quebecois friends and they don't go further than that. Because they change the subject, talk about something else. Then they don't get to know you beyond that. They don't feel attached to you. You don't get enough of a connection.

(Anna)

Similar to health and social service contexts, educational institutions were often experienced by participants as sites of surveillance and interrogation. Intersecting prejudices of age, race and status were experienced in ways that the participants described as devaluing their desires and erasing their personhood. In both cases, the young people disregarded and pushed back against attitudes and structures that they experienced as exclusionary and oppressive. Nevertheless, it is important to recognize that the culmination of these oppressive experiences have profound implications for people's psychological wellbeing and sense of trust and comfort when it comes to Quebec's education, health and social service systems.

Anna's quote above sheds light onto the often-reductive constructions young people with migrant backgrounds face in relation to their identity and experience. Anna described how such categorical understandings rendered her feeling as though people do not wish to see past this part of her reality and experience, and, as a result, she did not feel connected to some of her peers. In other words, the images many Canadians have of what constitutes an "immigrant" places constraint on the development of intimacy and genuine connection.

Furthermore, in the province of Quebec, participants also described experiences where they were met with impatience and sometimes mockery when trying to learn and speak the local French language:

Yes, in the school, it's going good, well. So, teachers are also nice, and students also, but sometimes, I don't know—most persons are getting mean when I speak in French, so they're going to do laughing, and I feel very sadness.

(Saddya)

Yeah, because I work on phones [as a telemarketer, part-time]. Like, sometimes, you talk with someone, they say: "You have an accent" . . . .Yeah, I understand, we have an accent, but they also have an accent. Like, they don't hear what you're saying, so they need another person. But there is a way, maybe, to say it politely. But last time, I got a customer, and she was like: "Ha-ha, you're funny". I'm like "Why?" "Why? You are funny. You have an accent and I can't understand you". She was like: "Next time, and make sure you write in your notes there. Next time, when you call, you have to ask a Quebecois [a native or inhabitant of Quebec, typically one who is French Canadian] to call me. I don't want any other person to call me, apart from a Quebecois."

(Jasmine)

While these quotes highlight the primacy of the French language in various educational and employment settings in the context of the province of Quebec, they also illustrate how participants were regularly confronted with experiences of exclusion, discrimination and racism. The challenges that come with learning a new language, in a completely new context, are compounded by the negative, often shaming, reactions many young people experience at the hands of their peers when attempting to learn and speak the language.

Specifically, most, if not all, young people resettling in the province of Quebec are placed in an intensive, 10-month long, *classe d'accueil*. Students in these classes are expected to learn French, and to become familiar with Quebecois values and customs, in order to successfully "integrate" into Quebec's school system and society, more broadly [30]. In this regard, learning French becomes a precursor for engaging in mainstream society [29]. However, young people from refugee backgrounds are often segregated from all other young people in the school they are attending, and remain together, as a group, for all other classes and school activities [29,30]. In this sense, social and linguistic "integration" is questionable. In one study of young people's experiences in a *classe d'accueil*, participants described how they were strictly forbidden from speaking any language but French, and were offered little individualised support while taking the course, and afterwards, when transitioning to mainstream classes [29].

Although young people may experience different forms of discrimination in this system, schools, nonetheless, appear to be important spaces for young people's wellbeing. For one, it was mainly through such spaces that young people were able to forge relationships, and connect with others with similar experiences, values and identities:

The first time I reached it it was very, very good for me to talk—to make communication; to make relationships with others.

(Obed)

You don't feel like, I'm the only person who became this way. Like, there are some other kids who are like me. Yeah, it gives you strength for like—okay [. . .] Yeah, so, it gives you—smile. We get together, we dance, we do whatever. You feel so—not alone.

(Jasmine)

And also in the class there were a lot of immigrants, there were a lot of Colombians. So during the break time, during the lunch time, we would always hang out together. We would speak Spanish, because we could always keep our culture, and we knew that we all have around the same values, the same...the same customs, you understand? [...] It felt good, because at least we could express ourselves. [. . .] we could at least talk to each other. Because it feels bad not to really have any friends in your classes. You feel discouraged, you feel depressed."

(Rodrigo)

These quotes shed light onto the integral role schools play as sites of human connection and belonging. Significantly, school offered participants the opportunity to forge new friendships and to connect through shared values, customs, languages and experiences. As the participants describe, this was particularly important in enhancing their emotional and social wellbeing, while counteracting some of the adverse effects of isolation and cultural invalidation.

Other participants reflected on the importance of key people in their respective school environments:

When I started school, the principal, she was a support to me... I don't know how to even describe it; the fact that she believed in and [...] I had teachers that encouraged me—because I was scared, I was scared to, to not be able to integrate and above all I was scared not to be able to succeed.

(Leah)

Participant: My class teacher, and my—I think, Kevin and Melissa. [. . .] I think Melissa and Kevin, they know perfectly. Because they are speak in Nepali also. And it's not perfect, but they are try to speak in Nepali. My class teacher, Melissa is too much intelligent . . . [she] speak in Nepali. Yeah, she's really good [. . .]

Interviewer: So, the fact that she was trying to speak Nepali is one of the things that made you feel safe?

Participant: Yeah.

These accounts demonstrate how young people's wellbeing and sense of comfort in school environments were also positively influenced by certain individuals in positions of authority, including teachers and principals. In both these testimonies, the participants describe how these people make them feel supported, and even safe in a completely unfamiliar system. The second quote, showing the exchange with the interviewer, sheds light onto the power of connecting with another through language, and the sense of security that this can instil in a young person in this context. Even if the teacher in this situation could not fluently speak the participant's mother tongue, the sheer effort reflects a form of relating that differs tremendously from more policing and prejudicial styles of relating. This reality stresses the importance of not assuming all formal education, health and social service settings as being inherently hostile. There are people, in all sorts of spaces, that are genuinely caring and that strive to empathize with, and do something about, the difficult positions that these young people find themselves in. These findings echo those identified in studies on young people from refugee backgrounds attending intensive English language schools or centres in Australia [9,13,17]. In these studies, young people remarked on the opportunities these spaces provided in terms of forging relationships with other young people with similar experiences and cultures, as well as in feeling supported and validated by teachers.

The critical consciousness and deep empathy of a few individuals, however, does not redress the participants' reported experiences of racism and social exclusion. These systemic issues left some participants feeling as though immigrant communities were being stripped of their language, culture and identity. This participant powerfully draws a parallel between cultural assimilation as experienced by Indigenous communities through the residential school system, and the assimilationist processes immigrants are subjected to, including *les classes d'accueil*, in the example of Quebec:

> *It's this issue of assimilation that I find not ... really not good. [...] The indigenous ... it's the Europeans really wanted to set up their own system. And they [the Indigenous] were... their children were obligated to go to these [residential] schools. And not speak their language, and they started drinking alcohol. It's not everyone, but they really have problems now [because of it]. So I tell myself: Immigrants could also lose their identity [like this?], because [...] the government controls, I find, they control a lot like what language you learn, what school you go to, what actions you take. If they aren't okay with the way you act like a good citizen, they're gonna stop you. So I find they control a lot. Or they say: 'Oh it's a free country, free religion" but me I'm not religious, but the law states where your religion could be and what location. And if there are religions that are not too ... that don't fall in the 'Western' category, well they find these...these loopholes to tell you: "No, this, these practices here, don't you do them." So it's really restrictive."*

(Anna)

People may argue against this point, emphasizing how the Quebecois are a linguistic and cultural minority in Canada and policies aimed to preserve the French language are integral in protecting the province's cultural identity. However, before anyone is to set forth an argument defending the assimilationist intent of Quebec's linguistic and cultural policies, a conversation needs to be had about Quebec's racially oppressive roots. The fervent call to safeguard Quebecois culture and identity elides the reality that various Onkwehonwe communities were the original people of this land (Onkwehonwe: Haudenosaunee word that in English translates to "the Original People" of this land) [37]. Moreover, it suggests that Quebec was a homogenous society, consisting mostly of white French settlers, when, in actuality, its populace has always been racially, culturally and linguistically diverse. Specifically, the myth of "homogeneity" ignores the central role the slavery of people of colour and Onkwehonwe, and the labour of various migrant communities, including the Chinese and Irish, played in the making of "Quebec" [37–40]. In this respect, in prioritizing the preservation of one culture, language and identity, the government, and its Quebecois subjects, are effectively endorsing a racial and cultural hierarchy.

The emphasis on cultural assimilation in Quebec's *classes d'accueil* appears particularly strong in comparison to similar programs in other white-settler nations. For instance, studies on intensive English language schools or centres in Australia reveal the tendency of such programs to adopt a more holistic and sociocultural approach to education and learning [9,13,14,17]. In such environments, young people's knowledge and values are recognised and celebrated. For instance, many in-class activities centre young people's identities, customs, and practices through the routine sharing of stories, language, food and festivals [13]. Often, loved ones and family members are welcomed into the classroom, effectively dismantling the school-home divide [13]. Although young people in such environments still report experiences of prejudice and exclusion, and, more generally, continue to contend with inequitable power relations [8,10–12,16], the prevailing cultural and racial hierarchy seems to be less rigid and more amenable to intercultural exchange and learning. Consequently, such contexts create powerful opportunities for teachers, and other persons in positions of authority, to connect to, experience and honour the humanity and lived realities of young people from refugee backgrounds. Likewise, by celebrating, rather than erasing, the customs and identities of these students, young people from refugee backgrounds are more likely to feel valued and validated, thereby nurturing the development of more trusting and healing relationships.

4. Solutions as Proposed by Participants

In addition to describing their experiences in formal settings, the participants were asked to suggest ways that current systems could be changed to better support young people from war-affected areas who have resettled in Canada. They were also encouraged to conceptualise new services and activities that they felt would better respond to their realities and needs.

Many participants called for institutional changes: Adjustments and improvements to the current systems in place. For instance:

Because [immigrants], to be honest, are more committed about doing something about their lives than anyone else. Because they've seen suffering. They see what it's like to be at the bottom of the barrel. They do not want to make mistakes so that their children suffer like they did. And if the government knows that, they'll be like, "Shucks, maybe we should invest more in these people because they are the ones were really going to build a foundation. [...] it is an investment to be involved in developing those people and not just letting them go and find a job in a factory when they have two or three children to raise, and thinking they will be able to raise their children. Really developing them in the sense that there's also that whole psychosocial counseling, things like that, that we spoke about, healthcare, education, as well. People who already have some kind of degree and need to get accreditation, Canadian-based, we should be involved in all that in this country.

(Andy)

In addition to *seeing* the humanity and immense commitment of immigrants in Canada, and ensuring their access to meaningful opportunities and support, this participant emphasises how people with immigrant and refugee backgrounds should play an active role in supporting the growth of migrant communities and in safeguarding their heritage:

Just because we are asking to be Canadian, doesn't mean that we want to no longer identify with our own heritage. There is still our own heritage that are holding onto. We still need some of it, you know. We still need that. Perhaps over many generations, everything is going to amalgamate. I don't know. But right here, right now, I think even for a sense of community, for sense of sanity, it's not a bad idea to make sure that the government is involved in some of the small community-building, in one way or another.

(Andy)

Specifically, in the context of schools, health clinics and hospitals, many participants emphasised the need to recognise and comprehensively address interpersonal and organisational forms of racism, xenophobia, and ignorance, more generally.

People don't trust the system. Maybe I don't trust it. I know a lot of people don't trust it. People don't even like to go to the hospital because they know. They don't have to tell them, "We don't want you here." Psychologically, the way they treat you, you feel it. That's all I can say. If you want me to study social work, bring more people who look like me. So when I talk to people who are like me they will feel comfortable telling me exactly what they're going through. People relate to people that they see can understand them. If they are Muslim, you talk to me, I don't have to judge you. I know exactly why you pray. But if you are not, and you've never been taught, you lock your mind to what you believe in, it's not going to work.

(David)

It would be good if the teachers would be more... more concerned [. . .] if they knew more like for example that there are people that lived through the war in their class, they would pay attention to these people, [and intervene] when comments go too far. Related to the war, related to... for example... the movies that they show us. Yes, maybe it's too violent. Maybe it's important to watch, but it's the comments that come afterwards. We could watch it, but it could be that someone actually lived through that. It's possible that...instead of reading, instead of finding it funny, to really take it seriously. And [. . .] to know how to respond to students. Like students that say: "Oh me I don't like immigrants because they will steal our jobs." The teacher would just sit there, he wouldn't say anything. To know how to respond like, what is the reality, what are the prejudices. I find there is a gap here for that.

(Anna)

This same participant advocates for programs that foster mutual understanding and connection between young people from refugee backgrounds and those from Quebec and that seek to dispel misconceptions and prejudices that they may hold towards one another.

Yes for sure that maybe [. . .] the [local] Quebecois students that are from here that...that like this...like being in charge of an immigrant in the beginning to explain the school to them, how it all works. "You have to go here, you have to go there" And that they act as a reference for you maybe. And maybe it becomes a friend. But more so that it is ....so that it has an impact on a wider level, I'm saying, like group gatherings with immigrants and people from here, and talk a bit about what they think about each other. Because for sure there are going to be prejudices on both sides [...] Other resources also. If there are people that are free to listen to us, or that know, that they come to talk to us, that they come to let us know that "We are here" that "We understand that you had to leave your country. If you need anything I am here for you." Because maybe they have the resources there, but they don't come and find you. So you don't know that you are supposed to go look for someone yourself.

(Anna)

The previous quote also highlights the need to have more *active* forms of support. Many of these young people are already struggling enough, and to have to struggle more in order to seek support for the struggles they are already dealing with seems nonsensical.

Other participants stressed the need to go beyond creating additional programs and adjusting what already exists, and suggested broad-based, transformative changes. These changes focused on Canada's national image and the hopeful promises it makes, as well as the dominant ways people interact and treat one another.

The truth has to be told to people. The system has to be honest with people. They give people so much hope that when they come to this country everything changes for them. Oh, your life will be perfect. And people come here, it's a constant battle. If you want to get help from CLSC you have to fight. If you want to get education, you have to fight. Why? I mean, you are the same people that say we want to accept you in society and making life more difficult for people. Come on. Is that fair? No. The Canadian government, whatever government it is [. . .] has the responsibility to treat people fairly. It's not a perfect system.

(David)

And it's a social issue I think. Because individualism is really strong in rich countries. [And if you don't live through something really intense with someone] [. . .] there is not that connection, there is not that way of listening [to each other]. So like I said its really in specific places, through things that you go through together, it's there that one can express themself. When you really know a lot about the person. And I want also to talk about the teachers. The teachers are always not ready for this, and it really doesn't help either. They aren't ready . . .

(Anna)

These accounts highlight how many young people from war-affected areas, over time, come to develop a sense of distrust, isolation and disconnection in a country whose national imagery poorly reflects the often divisive, and individualistic social relations that lie within. Canada is popularly touted as being an open, inclusive, supportive, welcoming and multicultural-loving space [37,38]. However, as described by participants throughout this paper, this does not seem to be an honest portrayal of young people's experiences in the province's public institutions, and within society, more generally.

The "taken for granted" legitimacy and inherent benevolence of current systems, and the well-intentioned people who staff them, is another major concern, along with the lack of diversity in these settings. As this participant describes:

But when [people] go in to seek help, [social workers] have to understand where [the person] comes from, what people talk about. It's not to follow a pre-scheduled way of asking questions without understanding the background. So, for me, it doesn't work. Refugees come here, go to prison [detention], and then after [detention] you have to work with social worker. You do what you have to do. Because [the social workers] they are part of the system. They follow a rigorous thing, instead of saying, look, maybe was that change this thing. I am not criticizing. I think having social work is a great thing, but there's something missing. [. . .] The only way social work can change in my opinion is to allow a lot of visible minority people who come from different background to do the work. [. . .] Because the thing is, if I'm talking to you, I already have in my mind, "well, this theory, she's going to follow the theory and this is the way it works."

(David)

Other participants advocated for the need to create more opportunities and spaces to foster a love of difference and human interconnectivity.

Yes in this moment we can say, maybe integration activities. Sometimes we see that organizations organize things for people to integrate, and share their culture [with others]. We always see positive things. Because unfortunately, no matter who or no matter what we always see first the negative things in other people. So that's why people that come are really distrusting of people that are not from the same culture or come from the same country.

(Rodrigo)

This participant insightfully draws attention to the ease with which people see the negative in one another, and from this, make grand generalizations that serve to divide, rather than unite, different communities. The distance such social relations engenders only reinforces the misconceptions different groups have of one another, thereby further fuelling prejudice and human disconnection. This cycle can be broken if intentional spaces are created where people can see the positive in one another and appreciate and honour difference and diversity. This participant provides an example of how such initiatives are already taking shape:

Yes let's take the example of the family's house, sometimes they organize... once a year or twice these intercultural activities or we see these dances, these songs from all these countries... Not all but definitely all the countries that the people come from. Do these dances and in there you see integration, you see that there are people interested in understanding new things... a new world that is outside of their own that they live in every day.

(George)

5. Conclusions

Young people from war-affected countries living in Quebec often find themselves at the intersection of complex forms of oppression that strongly shapes their emotional and mental wellbeing, and their experiences in various formalised spaces, including schools, hospitals and clinics. The hardships endured in their country of origin, compounded by the challenges that come with a new social, cultural, economic and political terrain, can profoundly influence young people's identity, sense of belonging and experiences of marginality. In other words, it is not strictly, nor necessarily, the violence that they may have experienced in their country of origin that adversely affects these young people's social, mental, emotional and material wellbeing, but more so the interaction between these past experiences, and the various, and often traumatizing, forms of injustice that many are faced with during and following resettlement.

The degree to which participants' identities and lived experiences are validated, understood and represented in these spaces may greatly influence how they choose to access and negotiate Quebec's public health and social services systems. In many cases, the prevailing biomedical model of disease may be out of sync with how participants conceptualise mental health and trauma. Systemic and interpersonal racism, Islamophobia and other forms of prejudice also appear to be central to people's experiences in these environments, threatening people's dignity and sense of security.

Participants' perspectives represented in this study shed light onto the varied difficulties and opportunities young people from war-affected countries negotiate upon resettlement. In particular, the participants' accounts can raise our awareness of how certain formal spaces of support are experienced as well as enhance our understanding of what is required in creating more inclusive, culturally-responsive, and meaningful services and programs.

By drawing on the framework of intersectionality, it is possible to disentangle the various, and interacting, dynamics that shape these young people's experiences within certain "formal" spaces. For one, the experiences of war, flight and resettlement are often foreign to those staffing these spaces. Many professionals may not know how to think, feel or act when listening to these young people describe the hardships they have endured. The experiences of flight, migration and resettlement further complicate professionals' capacity to connect with, and meaningfully support these young people. These realities can be, for many, unimaginable, and overwhelming for professionals. In addition, health and social service professionals are predominantly familiar with approaches to healing, and constructions of mental health, as conceptualized in the Global North, and may have a limited understanding of and appreciation for non-ethnocentric healing modalities [34]. As pointed out by some of the participants, "mental health" is often supported within the family or community, and not seen as an "issue" that warrants outside attention.

In addition to emphasising the power of *lived experience*, intersectionality stresses the need to critically consider how intersecting *marginal identities*, along the lines of race, citizenship status, class, religion and culture, are viewed and treated in these spaces. Experiencing prejudice first-hand, or expecting to experience prejudice, can profoundly affect young people's sense of security, comfort and belonging in health and social service settings. Being "othered" for wearing a hijab, for being black, and/or for being a migrant can make all the difference in a person's consideration of accessing, or outright avoiding, these environments.

In other words, when trying to understand young people's experiences and perceptions of these formal care settings, it is important to consider the *incongruity* between the histories, realities, life perspectives, "healing paradigms", and identities of these young people, and those of Quebec and Canadian-born professionals. Without striving for greater harmonisation between the norms, values, beliefs and perspectives of these spaces, and the lived experiences and identities of young people affected by war, health and social services risk exposing these young people to structural realities that may perpetuate oppressive and culturally imperialistic dynamics.

Schools also stand to benefit from seriously considering how current teaching methods, and the treatment of students with refugee backgrounds and from war-affected areas, serve to limit young people's capacity to learn, grow, and develop a sense of belonging. Professionals in these settings need to become more conscious of who is in their classrooms and to explore ways to nurture a learning culture that does not alienate or punish young people from war-affected countries for being who they are. To this end, professionals need to engage in an emotionally rigorous process of self-reflection in order to identify and change their own prejudices and biases against racialised people with refugee backgrounds. Strict segregation of immigrant and Quebec and Canadian-born young people through the *classes d'accueil* in the case of Quebec must also be addressed. This structure only reinforces divisiveness and thwarts opportunities for dialogue, intercultural exchange, belonging and human connection. Adopting a more holistic and sociocultural approach to education, similar to that being used in Australia, may be an important strategy for Quebec in this regard [13,17].

Understanding, through research and community engagement, the complex realities and needs of young people affected by war, and, in particular, their intersectional experiences of oppression, is imperative in order to promote and develop contextually-relevant and inclusive spaces of support in Quebec. Failing to do so will have profound implications for the wellbeing of young people from war-affected areas and their communities, and for Canadian society, as a whole. International migration stemming from war has been increasing globally, and at particularly high levels in Canada [4], and will continue to impact Canadian society. This underscores the importance of reconsidering the rudimentary tenants upon which various spaces of support and learning, namely schools and health care institutions, are built. Importantly, such challenges are not unique to Canada. Rather, they represent contemporary realities that continue to affect and have implications for host countries across the globe. By acknowledging and systemically addressing dominant social relations and structures that reinforce divisiveness as well as cultural and racial hierarchies, it is hoped that young people from war-affected areas will experience less "traumatising" forms of marginalisation, and instead experience more meaningful forms of support, healing and connection.

Author Contributions: Conceptualization, A.B. and M.D.; methodology, M.D.; formal analysis, M.D. and A.B.; data curation, M.D.; writing—original draft preparation, A.B. and M.D.; writing—review and editing, A.B. and M.D.; supervision, M.D.; project administration, M.D.; funding acquisition, M.D.

Funding: We are grateful to the Fonds de recherche du Québec—Société et culture (FRQSC) (grant #2013-SE-164334 and #2107-SE-196298) and the McGill Collaborative Research Grant (grant #120920) for their generous support of this research.

Conflicts of Interest: The authors declare no conflict of interest.

References

1. UNDP. *UNDP Youth Strategy 2014–2017: Youth Empowered as Catalysts for Sustainable Human Development*; UNDP: New York, NY, USA, 2014.
2. Stewart, J. *Supporting Refugee Children: Strategies for Educators*; University of Toronto Press: Toronto, ON, Canada, 2011.
3. Immigration, Refugees and Citizenship Canada. *2018 Annual Report to Parliament on Immigration*; Immigration, Refugees and Citizenship Canada: Ottawa, ON, Canada, 2018.
4. UNHCR. *Canada's 2016 Record High Level of Resettlement Praised by UNHCR*; UNHCR: Geneva, Switzerland, 2017.
5. Immigration, Refugees and Citizenship Canada. *2017 Annual Report to Parliament on Immigration*; Immigration, Refugees and Citizenship Canada: Ottawa, ON, Canada, 2017.
6. Denov, M.; Bryan, C. Unaccompanied Refugee Children in Canada: Experiences of Flight and Resettlement. *Can. Soc. Work Spec. Issue Settl. Integr. Newcom. Can.* **2010**, *12*, 67–75.

7. Denov, M.; Blanchet-Cohen, N. Trajectories of violence and survival: Turnings and adaptations in the lives of two war-affected youth living in Canada. *Peace Confl. J. Peace Psychol.* **2016**, *22*, 236–245. [CrossRef]
8. Riggs, D.W.; Due, C. Friendship, exclusion and power: A study of two South Australian schools with new arrivals programs. *Australas. J. Early Child.* **2010**, *35*, 73–80.
9. Due, C.; Riggs, D.W. Care for Children with Migrant or Refugee Backgrounds in the School Context. *Child. Aust.* **2016**, *41*, 190–200. [CrossRef]
10. Correa-Velez, I.; Gifford, S.M.; McMichael, C.; Sampson, R. Predictors of Secondary School Completion Among Refugee Youth 8 to 9 Years After Resettlement in Melbourne, Australia. *J. Int. Migr. Integr.* **2017**, *18*, 791–805. [CrossRef]
11. Correa-Velez, I.; Gifford, S.M.; McMichael, C. The persistence of predictors of wellbeing among refugee youth eight years after resettlement in Melbourne, Australia. *Soc. Sci. Med.* **2015**, *142*, 163–168. [CrossRef] [PubMed]
12. Correa-Velez, I.; Gifford, S.M.; Barnett, A.G. Longing to belong: Social inclusion and wellbeing among youth with refugee backgrounds in the first three years in Melbourne, Australia. *Soc. Sci. Med.* **2010**, *71*, 1399–1408. [CrossRef] [PubMed]
13. Due, C.; Riggs, D.W.; Augoustinos, M. Diversity in intensive English language centres in South Australia: Sociocultural approaches to education for students with migrant or refugee backgrounds. *Int. J. Incl. Educ.* **2016**, *20*, 1286–1296. [CrossRef]
14. Due, C.; Riggs, D.W.; Augoustinos, M. Experiences of School Belonging for Young Children with Refugee Backgrounds. *Educ. Dev. Psychol.* **2016**, *33*, 33–53. [CrossRef]
15. Peisker, V.C.; Tilbury, F. "Active" and "Passive" Resettlement: The Influence of Support Services and Refugees' own Resources on Resettlement Style. *Int. Migr.* **2003**, *41*, 61–91. [CrossRef]
16. Sampson, R.; Gifford, S.M. Place-making, settlement and well-being: The therapeutic landscapes of recently arrived youth with refugee backgrounds. *Health Place* **2010**, *16*, 116–131. [CrossRef] [PubMed]
17. Due, C.; Riggs, D.W.; Mandara, M. Educators' experiences of working in Intensive English Language Programs: The strengths and challenges of specialised English language classrooms for students with migrant and refugee backgrounds. *Aust. J. Educ.* **2015**, *59*, 169–181. [CrossRef]
18. Fraser, S.; Denov, M.; Guzder, J.; Bond, S.; Bilotta, N. Children of War: Quebec's Social Policy Response to Children and Their Families. *Int. J. Soc. Sci. Stud.* **2016**, *4*, 41. [CrossRef]
19. Blanchet-Cohen, N.; Denov, M.; Fraser, S.; Bilotta, N. The Nexus of War, Resettlement and Education: War-affected Youth's Perspectives and Responses to the Quebec Education System. *Int. J. Intercult. Relat.* **2017**, *60*, 160–168. [CrossRef]
20. Measham, T.; Guzder, J.; Rousseau, C.; Pacione, L.; Blais-McPherson, M.; Nadeau, L. Refugee Children and Their Families: Supporting Psychological Well-Being and Positive Adaptation Following Migration. *Curr. Probl. Pediatr. Adolesc. Health Care* **2014**, *44*, 208–215. [CrossRef] [PubMed]
21. Pacione, L.; Measham, T.; Rousseau, C. Refugee Children: Mental Health and Effective Interventions. *Curr. Psychiatry Rep.* **2013**, *15*, 341. [CrossRef] [PubMed]
22. Rousseau, C.; Gauthier, M.-F.; Benoît, M.; Lacroix, L.; Moran, A.; Viger Rojas, M.; Bourassa, D. Du jeu des identités à la transformation de réalités partagées: Un programme d'ateliers d'expression théâtrale pour adolescents immigrants et réfugiés. *Santé Ment. Au Qué.* **2006**, *31*, 135. [CrossRef]
23. Hadfield, K.; Ostrowski, A.; Ungar, M. What can we expect of the mental health and well-being of Syrian refugee children and adolescents in Canada? *Can. Psychol. Can.* **2017**, *58*, 194–201. [CrossRef]
24. Collins, P.H. *Black Feminist Thought: Knowledge, Consciousness, and the Politics of Empowerment*, 2nd ed.; Routledge: New York, NY, USA; London, UK, 2009.
25. Crenshaw, K. Mapping the Margins: Intersectionality, Identity Politics, and Violence against Women of Color. *Stanf. Law Rev.* **1991**, *43*, 1241. [CrossRef]
26. Hochreiter, S. Race, class, gender? Intersectionality troubles. *J. Res. Gend. Stud.* **2011**, *1*, 49–56.
27. Mehrotra, G. Toward a Continuum of Intersectionality Theorizing for Feminist Social Work Scholarship. *Affilia* **2010**, *25*, 417–430. [CrossRef]
28. Glaser, B.G.; Strauss, A.L. *The Discovery of Grounded Theory: Strategies for Qualitative Research*; Aldine Publishing Company: Chicago, IL, USA, 1967.
29. Allen, D. Who's in and who's out? Language and the integration of new immigrant youth in Quebec. *Int. J. Incl. Educ.* **2006**, *10*, 251–263. [CrossRef]

30. Steinbach, M. *Quand je sors d'accueil*: Linguistic integration of immigrant adolescents in Quebec secondary schools. *Lang. Cult. Curric.* **2010**, *23*, 95–107. [CrossRef]
31. Guzder, J.; Yohannes, S.; Zelkowitz, P. Helpseeking of immigrant and native born parents: A qualitative study from a montreal child day hospital. *J. Can. Acad. Child Adolesc.* **2013**, *22*, 275–281.
32. Thomson, M.S.; Chaze, F.; George, U.; Guruge, S. Improving Immigrant Populations' Access to Mental Health Services in Canada: A Review of Barriers and Recommendations. *J. Immigr. Minor. Health* **2015**, *17*, 1895–1905. [CrossRef] [PubMed]
33. Kirmayer, L.J.; Weinfeld, M.; Burgos, G.; du Fort, G.G.; Lasry, J.-C.; Young, A. Use of Health Care Services for Psychological Distress by Immigrants in an Urban Multicultural Milieu. *Can. J. Psychiatry* **2007**, *52*, 295–304. [CrossRef]
34. Whitley, R. Global Mental Health: Concepts, conflicts and controversies. *Epidemiol. Psychiatr. Sci.* **2015**, *24*, 285–291. [CrossRef]
35. Patil, C.L.; Maripuu, T.; Hadley, C.; Sellen, D.W. Identifying Gaps in Health Research among Refugees Resettled in Canada: Gaps in health research among refugees resettled in Canada. *Int. Migr.* **2015**, *53*, 204–225. [CrossRef]
36. Gadeberg, A.K.; Montgomery, E.; Frederiksen, H.W.; Norredam, M. Assessing trauma and mental health in refugee children and youth: A systematic review of validated screening and measurement tools. *Eur. J. Public Health* **2017**, *27*, 439–446. [CrossRef]
37. Thobani, S. *Exalted Subjects: Studies in the Making of Race and Nation in Canada*; University of Toronto Press: Toronto, ON, Canada, 2007.
38. Austin, D. Narratives of power: Historical mythologies in contemporary Québec and Canada. *Race Class* **2010**, *52*, 19–32. [CrossRef]
39. Cooper, A. *The Hanging of Angélique: The Untold Story of Canadian Slavery and the Burning of Montréal*; Harper Collins Publishers Inc.: Toronto, ON, Canada, 2006.
40. Choudry, A.; Mahrouse, G.; Shragge, E. Neither reasonable nor accommodating. *Can. Dimens.* **2008**, *42*, 16–18.

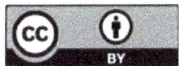

© 2019 by the authors. Licensee MDPI, Basel, Switzerland. This article is an open access article distributed under the terms and conditions of the Creative Commons Attribution (CC BY) license (http://creativecommons.org/licenses/by/4.0/).

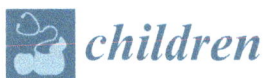

Review

Infectious Diseases among Refugee Children

Avinash K. Shetty

Department of Pediatrics and Office of Global Health, Wake Forest School of Medicine and Brenner Children's Hospital, Medical Center Blvd, Winston-Salem, NC 27157, USA; ashetty@wakehealth.edu; Tel.: +316-713-4500; Fax: +316-716-9699

Received: 1 November 2019; Accepted: 23 November 2019; Published: 27 November 2019

Abstract: In recent years, there has been a substantial increase in refugee and asylum-seeking adults, adolescents and children to high-income countries. Infectious diseases remain the most frequently identified medical diagnosis among U.S.-bound refugee children. Medical screening and immunization are key strategies to reduce the risk of infectious diseases in refugee, internationally adopted, and immigrant children. Notable infectious diseases affecting refugee and other newly arriving migrants include latent or active tuberculosis, human immunodeficiency virus type 1 (HIV), hepatitis B, hepatitis C, vaccine-preventable diseases, malaria, and other parasitic infections. The U.S. Centers for Disease Control and Prevention and the American Academy of Pediatrics have published guidelines for health assessment of newly arriving immigrant, refugee, and internationally adopted children. Although, data on the health risks and needs of refugee exists in some high-income countries, there is an urgent need to develop robust evidence-informed guidance on screening for infectious diseases and vaccination strategies on a broader scale to inform national policies. Innovative approaches to reach migrant communities in the host nations, address health and other complex barriers to improve access to high-quality integrated health services, and strong advocacy to mobilize resources to improve health, safety, and wellbeing for refugee children and their families are urgent priorities.

Keywords: refugee; migrant; children; infectious diseases; screening; immunizations

1. Introduction

In recent years, there has been a substantial increase in refugee and asylum-seeking adults, adolescents, and children to the European Union (EU)/European Economic Area (EEA) and the U.S. [1–5]. The Global Trends Report of the United Nations High Commissioner for Refugees (UNHCR) reported that by the end of 2017 approximately 68.5 million people were forcibly displaced across the globe, including 25.4 million refugees, 40 million internally displaced persons (IDPs), and 3.1 million asylum seekers [6]. By United Nations Children's Fund (UNICEF) estimates, 50 million children migrated across borders or suffered forced displacement within their own nations in 2015 [7]. More than 28 million children had to flee from their homes because of wars, violence, and insecurity [2]. Between 2010 and 2015, there has been a dramatic increase (75%) in the number of child refugees, with important implications for health care services [7].

Across Europe, children account for more than 30% of all asylum-seeking people [5]. In EU/EEA countries, an estimated 200,000 to 400,000 children sought asylum annually from 2015 to 2017; an additional 800,000 asylum-seeking children and adolescents arrived in 2015 to 2016 [1]. Asylum-seeking and refugee children from Syria, Afghanistan, and Iraq were the single largest group resettled in the EU/EEA in 2016 and 2017 [1,6]. Germany was the top country for asylum-seeking and refugee children in the EU and EEA followed by France, Greece, Italy, Austria, Sweden, the United Kingdom, Spain, and Switzerland [1].

The United States Citizenship and Immigration Services (USCIS), an agency nested under the Department of Homeland Security defines a *refugee* as an individual outside of his or her country of a nationality who is unable or unwilling to return to their native country because of persecution or a well-founded fear of persecution. An *asylee* is defined as an alien in the U.S. or at a portal of entry who is found to be unable or unwilling to return to native country because of persecution or a well-founded fear of persecution [3,8–11]. Refugee and asylum seekers are granted legal status in the U.S. Refugees typically undergo screening for resettlement outside of the U.S. whereas asylum seekers are physically in the U.S. at the time of their application submission [12]. Immigrant children are defined as children who are foreign-born, or children born in the U.S. who reside in a household with at least onee parent who is foreign-born [10].

In the U.S., from 2004 onwards, the number of refugee admissions per year has varied over the years, ranging from 41,094 to 74,602 annually, with 69,909 arrivals in 2013 [13]. In 2016, the number of refugee arrivals peaked at 84,994 followed by 53,716 admissions in 2017 [13]. Data from the U.S. State Department's Worldwide Refugee Admissions Processing System (WRAPS) indicates that the number of refugee admissions declined significantly to 22,491 in 2018 (a 58% decrease from 2017) [13] (Table 1).

Table 1. Top 10 Countries of origin with the highest refugee arrivals to the United States in 2017 and 2018.

2018		2017	
Country of Birth	No (%)	Country of Birth	No (%)
Dem. Rep. Congo	7878 (35.0)	Dem. Rep. Congo	9377 (17.5)
Burma	3555 (15.8)	Iraq	6886 (12.8)
Ukraine	2635 (11.7)	Syria	6557 (12.2)
Bhutan	2228 (9.9)	Somalia	6130 (11.4)
Eritrea	1269 (5.6)	Burma	5078 (9.5)
Afghanistan	805 (3.6)	Ukraine	4264 (7.9)
El Salvador	725 (3.2)	Bhutan	3550 (6.6)
Pakistan	441 (2.0)	Iran	2577 (4.8)
Russia	437 (1.9)	Eritrea	1917 (3.6)
Ethiopia	376 (1.7)	Afghanistan	1311 (2.4)

Data from [13].

During 1 October 2018 through to 30 April 2019, approximately 15,000 refugees were re-settled in the U.S.; of these, women and children aged less than 14 years represented 58% (8521) of refugee arrivals from the top five countries (Democratic Republic of Congo, Burma, Ukraine, Eritrea, and Afghanistan) [13]. In the first half of 2019, the top refugee-receiving states in the U.S. were Texas (9%, or 1389 individuals) and New York (6%, 932) followed by California (6%, 848) and Washington (6%, 827); other states including North Carolina (662), Ohio (651), Kentucky (649), Georgia (589), Michigan (584), and Arizona (536), accounted for 4% each. Overall, these 10 states represented 52% of all refugees resettled during the first half of 2019 [13]. Considerable variation exists among states by refugees' country of origin. For example, Burmese refugees historically were the single largest group resettled in the U.S. between 2007 through to April 2019 but were in the top group in only 19 U.S. states [13]. In contrast, 12 states, including California and Michigan, admitted more Iraqi refugees than any other country of origin during the past decade whereas Florida and Nevada have resettled more Cuba refugees than any other nationality group [13].

Newly arriving refugees and asylum seekers often arrive from low-income countries plagued by war and social conflicts, natural disasters, and economic challenges, and experience long journeys [14]. Poor health systems in the setting of conflicts can result in low vaccination coverage for children; in addition, history of vaccination and documentation of prior vaccine receipt is often incomplete [15,16]. In one cohort study of 2126 asylum-seeking children to Denmark, 30% were unimmunized based on the Danish immunization schedule [17]. In addition, the risk of communicable diseases is high given overcrowded circumstances during long migration journeys to Europe and other countries [18]. Refugees also face a myriad of challenges, including high mobility, poor living conditions, and barriers to access quality health care [10,19–21]. In addition, lack of interpretation services, cultural and language differences, limited health literacy and knowledge about health, lack of awareness regarding human rights, unfamiliar health systems, and lack of preparedness of health care providers in high-income countries to address the health and complex social issues of refugee populations further compound the problem [10,19,21].

Infectious diseases remain the most frequently identified medical diagnosis among refugee children arriving in the U.S. [22,23]. In addition, other key priority health conditions affecting refugee children is summarized in Table 2. Healthcare providers caring for refugee children must be aware of communicable diseases that are endemic to the refugee's country of origin. Priority infectious diseases affecting refugees and other newly arriving migrants to high-income countries include tuberculosis (TB) (active and latent), HIV, hepatitis B, hepatitis C, vaccine-preventable diseases (such as measles, mumps, rubella, diphtheria, tetanus, pertussis, and *Haemophilus influenzae* type b), and parasitic infections (such as strongyloidiasis and schistosomiasis) [4,22–24]. In the EU and EEA, infectious diseases are the most common cause of illness in migrant children living in refugee camps and other reception areas, including acute respiratory tract infections, outbreaks of vaccine-preventable diseases, such as measles, and skin infection (e.g., scabies, pediculosis); gastrointestinal infection (e.g., shigellosis); typhoid fever; hepatitis A; tuberculosis; and malaria [25,26].

Table 2. Key priority health issues in refugee children.

Health Issue	
Growth and Development Issues	• Various forms of Protein-Energy Malnutrition
Learning Difficulties	• Limited data available on educational outcomes
Vision and Hearing Impairments	• Refractory errors, presbyopia
Oral Health	• Dental caries
Vaccinations	• Risk for measles and other vaccine-preventable diseases
Nutritional Disorders	• Iron deficiency anemia • Micronutrient deficiency • Malnutrition • Vitamin D deficiency
Mental Health	• Depression • Anxiety • Posttraumatic stress disorder
Toxin Exposure	• Lead • Environmental pollution • Prenatal exposure to alcohol
Infectious Diseases	• Tuberculosis • Hepatitis A, B, C • Syphilis • Vaccine preventable diseases • Intestinal and tissue parasites *Giardia intestinalis, Cryptosporidium* species, *Ascaris lumbricoides, Trichuris trichura, Entamoeba histolytica,* hookworm, Schistosomiasis and Strongyloidiasis • Chagas Disease (American Trypanosomiasis)

In this article, we discuss the priority infectious disease affecting refugee children, review guidelines for evaluation and screening tests, and address preventative measures through immunizations.

2. Evaluation and Screening for Priority Infectious Diseases

Medical screening and immunization are key strategies to reduce the risk of infectious diseases in refugee, internationally adopted, and immigrant children [23,27–29]. The U.S. Immigration and Nationality Act (INA) mandates a medical screening examination performed by a designated civil surgeon and panel physicians for all refugees to identify inadmissible health conditions (e.g., imported communicable diseases). Inadmissible infectious diseases include: A) Communicable diseases of public health significance: Active tuberculosis (TB), syphilis (infectious stage), gonorrhea, and leprosy (infectious stage); B) communicable diseases that are listed as quarantine diseases in a presidential executive order: Cholera, diphtheria, plague, smallpox, yellow fever, viral hemorrhagic fevers, severe acute respiratory syndrome (SARS), and influenza caused by novel or re-emergent influenza (pandemic flu); and C) other infectious diseases designated as public health emergencies of international concern to the World Health Organization (WHO): Polio, smallpox, severe acute respiratory syndrome (SARS), influenza, and Ebola [12,29].

Compared to internationally adopted children, refugee children often undergo general medical screening (including a physical examination) in an organized fashion before the issue of an emigration visa pre-arrival in the U.S. [27–32]. Screening tests performed for U.S.-bound refugee children include serologic testing for syphilis, and tuberculin skin test or interferon gamma-release assay (child ages 2–14 years), and chest X-ray (for all applicants aged 15 years and older). In this setting, screening tests are often reliable since the screening process is coordinated by established reputable organizations [27]. In addition, access to primary prevention strategies, including immunizations, vitamin supplementation, and dental care, is generally more consistent with refugee children compared to internationally adopted children [27]. Certain tropical infections (e.g., malaria, filariasis, typhoid fever, schistosomiasis) are more frequently encountered in refugee children compared to internationally adopted children from countries outside sub-Saharan Africa [27].

The examination site and location is overseas for U.S.-bound immigrants and refugees and performed by panel physicians. A panel physician is a physician located outside the U.S, and authorized to conduct pre-immigration medical screening (for those individuals who apply for immigrant or refugee status prior to arrival in the U.S.). The U.S. Department of State selects the panel physicians. The U.S. Centers for Disease Control and Prevention (CDC)'s Division of Global Migration and Quarantine (DGMQ) provides technical instructions to civil surgeons and panel physicians who perform the mandated medical examinations for migrants [29]. The medical examination consists of a history and physical examination; laboratory screening tests for Tuberculosis (TB), syphilis, and gonorrhea; assessment of immunization status; diagnosis of mental health problems posing a danger to self or others; screening for substance abuse; and vaccinations for immigrants [33]. In addition, the CDC also provides pre-departure medical screening guidelines and health interventions for refugees based on risk in the country of origin, fitness to fly, and availability of resources and logistical support [29,34].

The U.S. CDC has published guidelines for the U.S. domestic medical examination for newly arriving refugees. [31]. Federal regulations do not require repeat medical screening examination for refugees upon arrival in the U.S. However, the Department of Health and Human Services recommends that all refugees have a post-arrival comprehensive assessment of health status and review of vaccinations by any qualified health care provider. The domestic medical assessment usually occurs 1 to 3 months after arrival as a coordinated effort between resettlement volunteer agencies and state public health departments [29]. Physician(s) at health departments who fulfill the legal requirements of a civil surgeon may participate in physical examination and vaccination assessment of refugees. A civil surgeon is a licensed U.S. physician with more than 4 years of experience and authorized by U.S. Citizenship and immigration Services (USCIS) to perform medical examinations [35]. CDC's post-arrival guidelines for refugee screening are available at [31]. Health care providers are encouraged to review site-specific clinical protocols via their local or state health department [29]. In addition, health profiles of diverse U.S.-bound refugee populations are maintained and updated by the CDC/Division of Global Migration and Quarantine (DGMQ) to inform health care providers regarding common health issues of newly arriving refugee groups [29].

The American Academy of Pediatrics recommends medical screening for all newly arrived refugee children and linkage to primary care as soon as possible after arrival [28]. The American Academy of Pediatrics (AAP) immigrant child health toolkit is a valuable resource for pediatricians caring for immigrant, refugee, and internationally adopted children [10,11,36]. The components of the AAP immigrant child health toolkit comprises of: Key facts, clinical care (e.g., medical screening, treatment recommendations for newly arrived immigrant children), mental and emotional health, access to health care and public benefits, immigration status and related concerns, state legal resources for immigrant children and families, and advocacy [10,36]. Screening tests for evaluation of common infectious diseases in refugee children are depicted in Table 3 [23,29]. The resources for clinicians caring for refugee children are summarized in Table 4.

Table 3. Screening tests for infectious diseases in refugee children, international adoptees, and immigrant children in the U.S. [23].

Disease	Screening Test	Comments
HIV	Serology (HIV 1 and 2)	Virologic tests (HIV DNA or RNA PCR) for children up to 18 months of age
Hepatitis A	Serology	
Hepatitis B	Serology	
Hepatitis C	Serology	
Syphilis	Serology	Nontreponemal tests (e.g., RPR, VDRL, or ART) Treponemal tests (e.g., MHA-TP, FTA-ABS, CIA, or TPPA)
Tuberculosis	TST or IGRA £ Chest X-ray *	• Medical History and Physical Examination • Sputum smears and cultures for individuals with an abnormal chest radiograph • Drug susceptibility testing for individuals with positive TB cultures • Completion of directly observed treatment prior to immigrant for individuals with pulmonary disease
Intestinal Parasites	Stool examination	Three specimens on separate days with requests for *Cryptosporidium* and *Giardia* species testing
Tissue Parasites:		
Schistosomiasis spp., *Strongyloides* spp., *Toxocara canis* Lymphatic filariasis €	Serologic testing	Screening for tissue parasites suggested in children with eosinophilia (absolute eosinophil count >450 cells/mm^3) and negative stool ova and parasite examination

Abbreviations: HIV, human immunodeficiency virus; IGRA, interferon-gamma release assay; PCR, polymerase chain reaction; TST, tuberculin skin test; £ IGRA-based TB testing has replaced TST in the 2017 Tuberculosis Technical Instructions (TBTI) for all applicants aged 2–14 years of age in high burden countries (WHO-estimated TB incidence rate of ≥20 cases per 100,000 population). * Chest X-ray is recommended for TB screening for all applicants aged 15 years and older. € Screen for lymphatic filariasis in children aged >2 years from endemic countries.

Table 4. Professional society and organizations with key resources for clinicians caring for immigrant, refugee, and internationally adopted children.

American Academy of Pediatrics (AAP)	• AAP Immigrant Child Health Toolkit
Canadian Collaboration for Immigrant and Refugee Health (CCIRH)	• Refugee health e-Learning, Evidence-based guidelines
lefts for Disease Control (CDC)	• Medical examination of refugees and immigrants, Refugee health guidelines and profiles, Laws and Regulations
International Organization for Migration (IOM)	• World Migration Report, Migration Profiles, Situation Reports
Minnesota Department of Health (MDH)	• left of Excellence in Refugee Health, Online interactive tool for CDC's domestic health screening guidance for individual refugees
Refugee Health Technical Assistance left (RHTAC)	• Best Practices for Communication to Refugees through Interpreter, Refugee suicide prevention training toolkit, Community Dialogue
United Nations Children's Fund (UNICEF)	• Research and reports, Stories from the field,
United Nations High Commissioner for Refugees (UNCHR)	• Global Report, Asylum Resources, Protection Manual
World Health Organization (WHO)	• Global Action Plan for promoting the health of refugees and migrants, Migrant Clinicians Network

2.1. Human Immunodeficiency Virus Type 1 (HIV)

HIV remains a major global public health challenge in many countries and disproportionately affects key vulnerable populations such as young men, women and children. Sub Saharan Africa bears the brunt of the HIV pandemic.

In 2018, 37.9 million (32.7 million–44.0 million) people worldwide were living with HIV including 1.7 million (1.3 million–2.2 million) children (<15 years) [37]. An estimated 20.6 million (18.2 million–23.2 million) people living with HIV reside in eastern and southern Africa [37]. From 1999 through to 2006, migrants, predominantly from sub-Saharan Africa, accounted for over half of people living with HIV in the 27 European Union countries [38].

The prevalence of HIV infection in newly arrived migrant children depends on the risk factors from their countries of origin (such as prevalence of maternal HIV infection and risk of mother-to-infant HIV transmission, maternal drug use, receipt of blood products) [5,23]. Studies from Germany, Italy, and Canada have documented an HIV prevalence of 0.4% to 2% among migrant children [39–41].

From 2010, routine HIV testing as part of the medical evaluation for immigration is not required for refugees and immigrants prior to arrival in the U.S. [28]. However, HIV testing is recommended for individuals who are diagnosed with TB disease as part of their medical outside of the U.S. After arrival in the U.S. the CDC recommends HIV testing for refugees aged 13 through to 64 years; HIV testing is encouraged for children aged younger than 13 years and adults older than 64 years [42]. Many factors determine the need to routinely screen for HIV infection in newly arrived migrant children in the U.S., including history, risk factors, physical examination findings, and HIV prevalence in the country of origin [23]. Some experts suggest that HIV testing may be indicated for most immigrant children [43].

Refugee children of any age with clinical suspicion for HIV should undergo testing. In infants and children younger than 18 months of age, virologic tests (HIV DNA or RNA assays) are recommended to screen for HIV infection since HIV antibody tests are unreliable due to the persistence of transplacental acquired maternal antibodies [23]. In contrast, in children aged 18 months and older, the diagnosis of HIV infection can be made by serology. If the diagnosis of HIV infection is confirmed by two-tier testing, referral to a pediatric infectious disease specialist for appropriate treatment and further evaluation is recommended [23].

2.2. Tuberculosis

Migrants often arrive from countries with a high incidence of TB [5,44]. In addition, the long travel and housing in overcrowded settings during re-settlement increases the risk of exposure to TB [45]. Classic symptoms of TB disease in children include fever, weight loss, and chronic, non-remitting cough. The most common forms of TB disease in children are pulmonary disease (hilar and mediastinal adenopathy, parenchymal disease) followed by extrapulmonary disease (tuberculous lymphadenopathy, meningitis, military disease). Compared to adults, extrapulmonary TB is more common in children [46]. Infants and young children are at higher risk of TB disease and progression to severe forms (such as tuberculous meningitis and military TB) following infection (latent disease) [46]. Therefore, screening for latent TB infection and early diagnosis and treatment of TB disease is crucial to reduce morbidity and mortality [47]. Studies from EU/EEA have reported a higher incidence of active TB is higher in migrant children compared with non-migrant children [5,48,49]. In one study from Germany, of 968 asylum-seeking children screened for TB, 66 (6.8%) children were diagnosed with TB infection (58 latent TB infection, 8 active TB) [48]. Studies report that approximately 1% of migrant children have evidence of active TB; rates up to 8% have been reported among newly arrived refugee children in the U.S. [50–54].

The U.S. revised pre-departure TB screening guidelines for immigrants in 2007 followed by complete implementation on a country-by-country basis in 2013 [29] (Table 3). Screening tests for TB are determined by the age of the child and HIV status and include the tuberculin skin test (TST) and interferon gamma-release assay (IGRA), chest radiograph, sputum smear, and culture and drug susceptibility testing [12,23,29,54]. A TST measurement of 10 mm or more of induration is considered positive (regardless of prior receipt of the Bacillus Calmette–Guérin (BCG) vaccine) whereas a TST induration of 5 mm or more is considered positive in children with HIV infection, exposure to a patient with active TB contact, or presence of symptoms and signs of TB [23].

In the 2007 U.S. CDC Tuberculosis Technical Instructions (TBTI), chest X-ray is the recommended test for TB screening for all U.S.-bound refugee and immigrants aged 15 years and older; for those with abnormal chest radiographs, symptoms or signs of TB disease, or known HIV infection, further evaluation with three sputum smear plus three cultures for Mycobacterium TB with drug susceptibility testing is recommended [54]. In addition, for all applicants aged 2 to 14 years of age in high-burden countries (WHO-estimated TB incidence rate of ≥20 cases per 100,000 population), screening with TST or IGRA was recommended; for those with positive tests, chest X-ray is recommended [54]. For refugee and immigrant children aged ≤2 years of age, no screening test is recommended (unless the child has symptoms or signs of TB or known active TB adult contact or HIV infection).

Based on 2007 TBTI, children aged 2 to 14 years with a positive TST or IGRA but negative chest X-ray or other evaluation for TB were classified as latent TB infection (LTBI). Children with LTBI can arrive in the U.S. without prior treatment but are recommended to undergo repeat evaluation for TB upon arrival [54]. Evaluation of children with LTBI found high rates of incomplete therapy in conjunction with overdiagnosis based on positive TST tests overseas but negative IGRA after arrival in the U.S. Therefore, IGRA-based TB testing has replaced TST in the 2017 U.S. CDC-based Tuberculosis Technical Instructions (TBTI) for all applicants aged 2 to 14 years of age in high-burden countries (WHO-estimated TB incidence rate of ≥20 cases per 100,000 population) [29,54].

Many refugee children would have received the Bacillus Calmette–Guérin (BCG) vaccine, a common practice in countries with a high incidence of TB. The BCG vaccine has limited efficacy in the prevention of pulmonary TB but is around 80% effective in preventing serious, potentially fatal, disease, such as military TB and TB meningitis in children. Prior receipt of the BCG vaccine is not a contraindication for TST. However, TST may be false positive in children who have previously received the BCG vaccine [55]. In such instances, obtaining an IGRA may be helpful in determining the cause of a "positive" TST (latent TB infection versus BCG vaccine-related) [56]. False-negative TST or IGRA results may be encountered in refugee children who are anergic due to a variety of reasons, such as malnutrition, stress, and untreated HIV infection. Studies have shown that screening for latent TB infection in young migrant children from high incidence countries is also cost effective [57–59].

Any child with a positive TST or IGRA warrants further evaluation by performing a physical examination and obtaining a chest radiograph to exclude TB disease. Given the high prevalence of drug-resistant TB in many countries, efforts to isolate the pathogen via obtaining sputum samples (via early morning gastric aspirates or sputum induction) for drug susceptibility testing is crucial [12,23]. Applicants diagnosed with active TB must complete treatment via directly observed therapy prior to arrival in the U.S. [29].

2.3. Syphilis

Refugee children and adolescents may be exposed to sexual violence and abuse before resettlement. However, data on the prevalence of syphilis in migrant children is limited [5]. One study from the U.S. has reported a relatively high rate of syphilis seropositivity in refugees arriving from the African region (874 cases out of 233,446 screened corresponding to 373 cases per 100,000); adolescents and young adults from aged 15 to 24 years accounted for 101 (11.6%) of all cases of syphilis seropositivity [60].

Refugee children aged 15 years and older undergo routine screening for syphilis using a two-stage serologic testing procedure at a specified in-country reference laboratory prior to arrival in the U.S. [31]. The initial screening is performed using non-treponemal tests (e.g., Venereal Disease Research Laboratory (VDRL)) or rapid plasma regain (RPR), and if found reactive are confirmed with an appropriate treponemal test. Refugees with reactive test results have to complete treatment for syphilis in accordance with the CDC's sexually transmitted guidelines prior to arrival in the U.S. [61].

After resettlement, screening for syphilis (and other sexually transmitted infections) is recommended if there is a concern for congenital syphilis, sexual abuse, or positive maternal syphilis serology. Children with reactive syphilis serology should be referred to pediatric infectious disease specialists or health care providers at the local health departments to confirm the diagnosis, disease staging, and treatment; in addition, infection due to other treponemal subspecies (e.g., yaws, bejel, and pinta) must be excluded [23].

2.4. Hepatitis A

Hepatitis A virus (HAV) is an endemic disease in many countries of origin of migrant children. Outbreaks of HAV have occurred among refugee children from Syria, Afghanistan, and Iraq living in hosting facilities in Greece, Germany, and other countries [62]. The spread of HAV occurs via the fecal–oral route and predominantly affects school-aged children 5 to 9 years of age [23,63]. Serologic testing of children at the time of the initial visit to the health care provider can determine acute infection [Immunoglobulin (Ig)M antibody to HAV] from immune status (total HAV IgM and IgG). Most children may have natural immunity from prior HAV infection acquired at their country of origin whereas others may be non-immune and candidates for vaccination against HAV. In a study in refugees and asylum seekers in Germany on the immunity against hepatitis A-E viruses, 81% of refugee minors were immune, which corresponds to the high anti-HAV seroprevalence rates in patients from Sub-Saharan and Northern Africa, and from the Middle East [64]. The U.S. CDC and AAP recommends the hepatitis A vaccine as part of the routine immunization schedule for all children aged 1 year and older without evidence of immunity [23].

2.5. Hepatitis B

Hepatitis B virus (HBV) infection is a serious public health challenge in many countries, with an estimated 257 million people living with chronic HBV infection worldwide [65]. The Pacific Islands, Southeast and East Asia, Africa, Middle East, and Central and Eastern Europe have the highest incidence of HBV [66]. The transmission of HBV occurs via infected blood or body fluids. The primary routes of transmission of HBV are vertical (mother-to-child) and horizontal early childhood transmission, resulting in the most chronic infection [67]. The reported prevalence of positive HBsAg was 15% in migrants from sub-Saharan Africa resettled in Spain and up to 10% among undocumented migrants in Italy [68–70].

Perinatal HBV infection results in chronic liver disease in 90% of children; early mortality is noted in 25% of untreated children with chronic liver disease due to HBV-related cirrhosis and hepatocellular carcinoma [71]. Universal hepatitis B immunization at birth and in infancy is the key strategy for global elimination of HBV infection, and has been highly effective in reducing new vertical infections [72]. In many endemic countries for HBV, infants do not receive the HBV vaccine at birth or early infancy. Therefore, serologic testing to screen for chronic HBV infection using HBsAg is recommended for all immigrant, refugee, and internationally adopted children regardless of immunization status [23]. Studies have shown that migrant serologic screening for HBV infection is also cost effective [73,74].

Local or state health departments must be notified of positive HBsAg results. Children with positive HBsAg test results should be re-tested and additional serologic markers to HBV core Ag performed to differentiate acute (positive IgM anti-HBc) from chronic HBV infection (negative IgM anti-HBc, positive total anti-HBc, and persistence of HBsAg for at least 6 months). [23]. Children diagnosed with chronic HBV infection must be referred to a pediatric infectious disease specialist for further evaluation and management.

2.6. Hepatitis C

The burden of hepatitis C virus (HBV) infection is high in China, Russia, and South East Asia, with an estimated prevalence of 0.15% in children 1 to 19 years of age, resulting in 3·5 million people living with HCV infection (95% CI 3.1–3.9 million). [75]. HCV infection is usually asymptomatic in the pediatric age group; in contrast to chronic HBV infection, complications of cirrhosis and hepatocellular carcinoma are unusual.

Serologic testing to screen for HCV is recommended for all immigrant, refugee, and internationally adopted children [23]. Initial screening tests for HCV infection include obtaining a serum enzyme immunoassay (ELISA). However, in children up to 18 months of age, a positive ELISA may reflect passively transferred maternal antibody to HCV. Further evaluation with a recombinant immunoblot assay or polymerase chain reaction for HCV should be considered for confirmation of HCV infection following a positive ELISA test result. Children with HCV infection must be referred to a pediatric infectious disease specialist for further evaluation and long-term follow-up [23].

2.7. Vaccine-Preventable Diseases

The high burden of vaccine-preventable diseases among migrant children compared with non-migrant children underscores the need for timely vaccination in this vulnerable population [76–80]. Despite the recommendations for age-appropriate vaccinations for migrant children with absent or uncertain immunization records, studies have shown that migrants in the EU are not up to date on vaccinations [81,82]. A cohort study from Denmark showed that 30% of asylum-seeking children were not up to date on vaccinations in accordance with national guidelines [17]. In another report from Sweden, measles seroimmunity gaps were noted in newly arrived adult immigrants from certain European regions and Russia [83]. An outbreak of measles was reported in 2017 from Minnesota, U.S., which predominantly affected children of Somali descent [84]. Another study among Somali refugees in Minnesota reported that 18% of the study participants were seronegative for varicella, underscoring the need for enhanced education to improve varicella vaccination rates in these at-risk communities [85]. Another study from Minnesota indicated that childhood vaccination coverage at 36 months was 44% in children born to mothers from Somalia compared with 77% in children born to mothers from Central and South America [86]. Declines in MMR vaccine coverage secondary to vaccine safety concerns have been reported in children born to Somali parents in Minnesota compared with children born to non-Somali parents [87]. In conflict settings, outbreaks of polio and other VPDs are a major cause of morbidity and mortality, with the potential to spill over to neighboring nations [88–91].

2.8. Intestinal and Tissue Parasites

Stool examinations for ova and parasites performed at a laboratory by those with expertise in parasitology may yield a parasite in 15% to 35% of migrant children [23]. The prevalence of intestinal parasitic infection varies based on country of origin and age. Commonly diagnosed intestinal parasitic infections are *Giardia intestinalis*, *Cryptosporidium* species, *Ascaris lumbricoides*, and *Trichuris Trichura* followed by *Strongyloides stercoralis*, *Entamoeba histolytica*, and hookworm [92]. Newly arrived migrants with complaints of diarrhea should be screened for infection due to *Cryptosporidium* species and other invasive bacterial pathogens, including *Salmonella*, *Shigella*, *Camplylobacter*, and diarrheagenic *E. coli* species (including Shiga toxin-producing *E. coli*).

Since 1999, the Centers for Disease Control and Prevention (CDC) recommended a single dose of presumptive albendazole treatment for intestinal parasites, administered overseas for U.S.-bound refugees. This approach has resulted in a significant decline in the prevalence of intestinal helminths (from 22.5% to 7.5%) among newly arrived refugees from Africa and Southeast Asia [93]. The CDC has published treatment guidelines for intestinal parasites based on prior receipt of presumptive albendazole therapy in U.S.-bound refugee children [34]. A total of three stool specimens collected on different days for ova and parasites is recommended for the screening of intestinal parasitic infection among all immigrant, refugee, and internationally adopted children arriving in the U.S. regardless of nutritional status or presence of symptoms. [23]. However, data from Germany indicate no evidence of the benefit of routine stool screening to detect intestinal parasites among refugee minors [94]. Tissue-invasive parasitic infections, such as schistosomiasis and strongyloidiasis, must be included in the differential diagnosis of recently arrived immigrants and refugee children with unexplained eosinophilia (defined as an absolute eosinophil count greater than 450 cells/µL with negative stool testing for ova and parasites) [23,28,95,96]. Around 30 to 250 million people have schistosomiasis and strongyloidosis in endemic countries [4].

A high prevalence of schistosomiasis (9% to 60%) has been reported among adolescent migrants from sub-Saharan Africa re-settled in Germany, Switzerland, Spain, and Canada [53,95,97,98]. *Schistosoma mansoni* and *S. haematobium* are the two primary species of Schistomas causing intestinal and genitourinary disease, respectively. Serious long-term complications of untreated schistosoma infection include hepatic cirrhosis, portal hypertension, bladder and ureter fibrosis, hydronephrosis, and bladder cancer [99,100]. Serologic testing for schistosoma is very sensitive and is recommended for all migrant children from endemic countries who have evidence of eosinophilia, negative stool ova and parasite examination, and exclusion of common infections associated with eosinophilia [23,31,33]. However, an eosinophil count may not be a good screening parameter for schistosomiasis and universal serological screening might be more beneficial; in one study, 25% of refugees from sub-Saharan Africa had schistosomiasis but only 7.7% had a high eosinophil count [98]. The positive- and negative-predictive value of the eosinophil count is poor and therefore, some experts suggest schistosomiasis serology in all migrant children from high-endemic countries, regardless of their eosinophil count [23]. In some settings in the EU, circulating-cathodic-antigen (CCA) rapid point-of-care assay are available [101]. In refugee children aged 2 years and older with eosinophilia, serologic testing for lymphatic filariasis is a consideration if they have arrived from countries endemic for lymphatic filariasis [23,31,33].

Stronglyloides stercoralis is an intestinal parasitic disease, prevalent in many parts of the world, with a propensity to cause life-threatening disease, especially in immunocompromised hosts after a prolonged period of subclinical infection [102]. Serologic testing for strongyloides is recommended for all refugee children with unexplained eosinophilia regardless of country of origin [23,31,33,95].

2.9. Chagas Disease (American Trypanosomiasis)

Chagas disease, also known as American trypanosomiasis, is a zoonotic tropical infection caused by a protozoan parasite *Trypanosoma cruzi*. Most infections in humans occur via vector-borne transmission through infected triatomine insects in endemic locations; other routes of transmission include vertical from mother to baby or receipt of blood transfusion in a country with endemic Chagas disease. The disease is endemic in Mexico, and Central and South America and estimated to affect 6 to 8 million people in the Americas, including 326,000 to 347,000 in the U.S. [103]. Following a prolonged asymptomatic phase, chronic CD can result in serious cardiac and gastrointestinal complications in approximately 30% to 40% of infected patients. Cases of CD have been reported from migrants arriving from Latin America to the U.S. and Canada, but the disease seems to be rare in Europe, although the diagnosis may be missed due to a lack of knowledge and awareness among patients and providers in non-endemic countries.

In suspected cases, the diagnosis is confirmed by serology by detection of IgG antibodies against *T. cruzi* utilizing at least two different assays (such as ELISA, indirect immunofluorescent, or indirect hemagglutination). Serologic screening for Chagas disease is only recommended for children older than 12 months due to the potential interference by the persistence of maternal antibody [23].

2.10. Malaria

Sub-Saharan Africa has the highest burden of malaria, with more than 90% of malaria cases and deaths, primarily in children aged less than 5 years [104]. The benefit of routine post-arrival screening for malaria in asymptomatic cases is unclear and not recommended given the limited sensitivity of diagnostic tests, such as blood films and rapid antigen tests [5,12].

U.S.-bound refugee children from sub-Saharan Africa that are endemic for *Plasmodium falciparum* malaria would have received pre-departure presumptive treatment with artesunate combination therapy unless contraindicated in certain specific groups (e.g., pregnant or lactating women, children with body weight less than 5 kg at time of departure). U.S.-bound refugee children from a malaria-endemic country or from sub-Saharan Africa who present with a febrile illness should be promptly evaluated to exclude malaria [105].

2.11. Other Infections

Other infectious diseases, especially of the skin, such as impetigo, candidiasis, tinea, scabies, and pediculosis are frequently diagnosed in refugee and internationally adopted children and adolescents, reflecting unhygienic living situations, overcrowding, and social marginalization [23,106]. Outbreaks of vaccine-preventable diseases (e.g., measles), and gastrointestinal and cutaneous infections have been reported in the early settlement period [107,108]. Health care workers must be aware of the clinical presentations of other tropical infectious diseases prevalent in the refugee country of origin, such as typhoid fever, Zika, cysticercosis, echinococcosis, leprosy, cutaneous diphtheria, chronic helminthiasis, and louse-borne relapsing fever [24,109].

3. Prevention

Vaccination Strategies

As part of the medical examination, all U.S.-bound refugees undergo an assessment of vaccine-preventable diseases (polio, tetanus, diphtheria toxoids, pertussis, *Haemophilus influenza* type b, rotavirus, mumps, measles, rubella, hepatitis A, hepatitis B, meningococcal disease, influenza, pneumococcus, and varicella). However, refugees and internationally adopted children can enter the U.S. with an incomplete immunization schedule. Based on the U.S. Immigration and Nationality

Act, there is no requirement for U.S.-bound refugees to meet immunization requirements. However, proof of immunization status is required for refugees already residing in the U.S. and applying for an adjustment of status for permanent residency, usually 1 year after arrival.

Clinicians should review immunization records, if available, to determine if the vaccine doses and intervals are consistent with the age-appropriate immunization recommendations of the U.S. Advisory Committee on Immunization Practices (ACIP) and other national guidelines [23,31,110–112].

An accurate assessment of immunization status in refugee children is challenging because of an unreliable history and uncertainty in the clinical diagnosis of vaccine preventable diseases (VPDs), such as measles, mumps, rubella, and varicella. Assessment of immunity against VPDs by measurement of antibody titers in refugees is limited. One study found that sero-testing for varicella immunity was more cost effective compared with universal administration of the varicella vaccine in refugee children [113]. Vaccination without obtaining serologic tests for VPDs may be a consideration in some settings since tests may be expensive, have a delayed turnaround time, and patients may be lost to follow-up due to re-location.

According to the U.S. Immigration and Nationality Act of 1996, for refugees with absent records or incomplete immunization status, a single vaccine dose in a series recommended by the U.S. Advisory Committee on Immunization Practices (ACIP) suffices for the immigration process, with a plan to complete the remaining doses in a series and catch-up vaccinations [23,31,113].

4. Knowledge Gaps, Research Agenda, and Future Directions

Public health programs are crucial for implementation of the screening and evaluation of migrants for infectious diseases. Historically, screening and quarantine procedures were performed utilizing port-of-entry strategies at the time of arrival of ships [114]. However, given the different routes of travel and dramatic increase of newly arriving migrants, the effectiveness of this strategy is limited [115]. For more than two decades, the U.S. Centers for Disease Control and Prevention's Division of Global Migration and Quarantine has implemented a health assessment framework (overseas screening, treatment, and immunization programs) to improve health for US-bound immigrants and refugees [29]. This program has had many successes, including decreased TB rates in the U.S., decreased transmission and importation of VPDs, reduction in morbidity from parasitic diseases, and reduced domestic healthcare costs [116].

Migrant health reviews from Canada indicate that disease risk is affected by many factors, such as gender, forced migration, and migrant country of origin, and provide important guidance to develop evidence-based evaluation and vaccination strategies [117]. Similar migrant health reviews from Ireland, Australia, and other countries have also provided evidence to inform public health policy and primary care assessments [114,115,117,118]. Data from the Migration Integration Policy Index health system survey indicate that evidence-based programs, guidelines, and policy for infectious disease, mental health, and maternal health, and chronic disease evaluation of migrants is limited and warrants further studies in many countries in Europe [4,119,120]. The cost effectiveness of the implementation of screening and treatment of latent TB infection and effectiveness to prevent active TB disease is an area of future research [121]. The development of evidence-based guidance for screening, treatment, and prevention of infectious diseases, including vaccine-preventable diseases, in newly arrived migrants is a major public health priority of the European Centre for Disease Prevention and Control (ECDC) [4,5].

The United Nations Convention on the Rights of the Child state that migrant children must receive the same standard of health care as received by the local population [122]. A recent review on migration and infectious diseases highlights the importance of screening programs tailored to various steps in the migratory pathway and improve access to care irrespective of the legal status of the individual [22]. However, engaging refugee and other migrant populations in health care and prevention services remains a challenge due to many barriers to accessing health care services, such as high rates of non-insurance, lack of health information, language and cultural differences, transportation issues, stigma, discrimination, and social isolation [10,123,124].

The reported outbreak of measles among Somali children in Minnesota who were not up to date on measles-mumps-rubella (MMR) vaccinations due to safety concerns (erroneous link to autism) highlights the need to develop enhanced community outreach and education with families and Somali community leaders to address vaccine hesitancy, provide health education, and improve vaccination rates [86]. Studies with a rigorous study design must be conducted to assess interventions to successfully implement vaccination programs for migrant populations [125,126]. In conflict zones and complex humanitarian emergency settings, the implementation of mass immunization campaigns has resulted in controlling the outbreaks of wild polio virus and circulating vaccine-derived poliovirus infections, suggesting that innovative approaches to vaccinate children on the move are needed [127,128]. Cost-effective interventions to address health care disparities and provide high-quality primary and secondary health care for large numbers of recently arrived migrants remains a major priority for many high-income countries [10,11,28,129–132].

An estimated 18 million children reside in the U.S. with at least one immigrant parent; 4.5 million children are U.S. citizens with mixed immigration status with at least one family member with undocumented status [133]. Recent changes in U.S. immigration policy related to unaccompanied children, family separation, and detention of people arriving from El Salvador, Honduras, and Guatemala at the Southern border of Mexico has been a major concern [134]. Strong advocacy efforts and policy statements by the American Academy of Pediatrics provide recommendations for the care of immigrant children following release from detention facilities to address medical and legal needs, education, and interpretation services. [135,136]. Increased funding in conjunction with multi-sector collaboration between governments, nongovernmental organizations, and local community agencies are needed to address the complex social, health, and economic needs of refugee and immigrant children and youth [137,138].

5. Conclusions

Infectious diseases often threaten the health of migrant populations and host communities. Key priority infectious diseases among refugee populations include tuberculosis, hepatitis B, and vaccine-preventable and parasitic diseases. Although data on the health risks and needs of refugee exists in some high-income countries, there is an urgent need to develop robust evidence-informed guidance on screening for infectious diseases and vaccination strategies on a broader scale to inform national policies. Innovative approaches to reach migrant communities in the host nations, address health and other complex barriers to improve access to high-quality integrated health services, and strong advocacy to mobilize resources to improve health, safety, and wellbeing of refugee children and their families are urgent priorities.

Author Contributions: Conceptualization, methodology, and writing, A.K.S.

Conflicts of Interest: The author declares no conflict of interest.

References

1. United Nations Children's Fund (UNICEF). *Latest Statistics and Graphics on Refugee and Migrant Children*; UNICEF: New York, NY, USA, 2018. Available online: http://www.unicef.org/eca/emergencies/refugee-andmigrant-children-europe (accessed on 19 July 2019).
2. United Nations Children's Fund (UNICEF). *Key Facts and Figures*; UNICEF: New York, NY, USA, 2018; p. 2. Available online: https://data.unicef.org/resources/children-move-key-facts-figures/ (accessed on 19 July 2019).
3. United States Department of Homeland Security. *Yearbook of Immigration Statistics: 2017*; U.S. Department of Homeland Security, Office of Immigration Statistics: Washington, DC, USA, 2018. Available online: https://www.dhs.gov/yearbook-immigration-statistics (accessed on 17 July 2019).

4. Pottie, K.; Mayhew, A.D.; Morton, R.L.; Greenaway, C.; Akl, E.A.; Rahman, P.; Zenner, D.; Pareek, M.; Tugwell, P.; Welch, V.; et al. Prevention and assessment of infectious diseases among children and adult migrants arriving to the European Union/European economic association: A protocol for a suite of systematic reviews for public health and health systems. *BMJ Open* **2017**, *7*, e014608. [CrossRef] [PubMed]
5. Schrier, L.; Wyder, C.; Del Torso, S.; Stiris, T.; von Both, U.; Brandenberger, J.; Ritz, N. Medical care for migrant children in Europe: A practical recommendation for first and follow-up appointments. *Eur. J. Pediatr.* **2019**. [CrossRef] [PubMed]
6. United Nations High Commissioner for Refugees (UNHCR). *Global Report 2017*; UNCHR: Geneva, Switzerland, 2017. Available online: http://www.unhcr.org/publications/fundraising/5b4c89bf17/unhcrglobal-report-2017.html (accessed on 17 July 2019).
7. United Nations Children's Fund (UNICEF). *Uprooted—The Growing Crisis for Refugee and Migrant Children*; UNICEF: New York, NY, USA, 2016; p. 3. Available online: https://www.unicef.org/publications/files/Uprooted_growing_crisis_for_refugee_and_migrant_children.pdf (accessed on 19 July 2019).
8. Passel, J.S. Demography of immigrant youth: Past, present, and future. *Future Child.* **2011**, *21*, 19–21. [CrossRef] [PubMed]
9. United States Citizenship and Immigration Services (USCIS). Available online: http://www.uscis.gov/tools/glossary (accessed on 15 July 2019).
10. Linton, J.M.; Choi, R.; Mendoza, F. Caring for children in immigrant families: Vulnerabilities, resilience, and opportunities. *Pediatr. Clin. N. Am.* **2016**, *63*, 115–130. [CrossRef] [PubMed]
11. Turner, C.; Ibrahim, A.; Linton, J.M. Clinical tools working at home with immigrants and refugees. *Pediatr. Clin. N. Am.* **2019**, *66*, 601–617. [CrossRef] [PubMed]
12. Waggoner-Fountain, L.A. Management of refugees and international adoptees. *Pediatr. Clin. N. Am.* **2017**, *64*, 953–960. [CrossRef]
13. U.S. Department of State. *Refugee Processing Center*; Department of State Bureau of Population, Refugees and Migration: Arlington, VA, USA, 2016. Available online: http://www.wrapsnet.org/admissions-and-arrivals (accessed on 17 July 2019).
14. Lori, J.R.; Boyle, J.S. Forced migration: health and human rights issues among refugee populations. *Nurs. Outlook.* **2015**, *63*, 68–76. [CrossRef]
15. Mipartrini, D.; Stefanelli, P.; Severoni, S.; Rezza, G. Vaccinations in migrants and refugees: A challenge for European health systems. A systematic review of current scientific evidence. *Pathog. Glob. Health.* **2017**, *111*, 59–68. [CrossRef]
16. Pavlopoulou, I.D.; Tanaka, M.; Dikalioti, S.; Samoli, E.; Nisianakis, P.; Boleti, O.D. Clinical and laboratory evaluation of new immigrant and refugee children arriving in Greece. *BMC. Pediatr.* **2017**, *17*, 132. [CrossRef]
17. Nakken, C.S.; Skovdal, M.; Nellums, L.B.; Friedland, J.S.; Hargreaves, S.; Norredam, M. Vaccination status and needs of asylum-seeking children in Denmark: A retrospective data analysis. *Public Health* **2018**, *158*, 110–116. [CrossRef]
18. Eichner, M.; Brockmann, S.O. Polio emergence in Syria and Israel endangers Europe. *Lancet* **2013**, *382*, 1777. [CrossRef]
19. Rechel, B.; Mladovsky, P.; Ingleby, D.; Mackenbach, J.P.; McKee, M. Migration and health in an increasingly diverse Europe. *Lancet* **2013**, *381*, 1235–1245. [CrossRef]
20. Febles, C.; Nies, M.A.; Fanning, K.; Tavernier, S.S. Challenges and strategies in providing home based primary care for refugees in the US. *J. Immigr. Minor. Health* **2017**, *19*, 1498–1505. [CrossRef] [PubMed]
21. Kadir, A.; Battersby, A.; Spencer, N.; Hjern, A. Children on the move in Europe: A narrative review of the evidence on the health risks, health needs and health policy for asylum seeking, refugee and undocumented children. *BMJ. Paediatr. Open* **2019**, *3*, e000364. [CrossRef]
22. Castelli, F.; Sulis, G. Migration and infectious diseases. *Clin. Microbiol. Infect.* **2017**, *23*, 283–289. [CrossRef]
23. American Academy of Pediatrics. Medical evaluation for infectious diseases for internationally adopted, refugee and immigrant children. In *Red Book: 2018–2021 Report of the Committee on Infectious Diseases*, 31st ed.; Kimberlin, D.W., Brady, M.T., Jackson, M.A., Long, S.S., Eds.; American Academy of Pediatrics: Elk Grove Village, IL, USA, 2018; pp. 176–185.
24. Eiset, A.H.; Wejse, C. Review of infectious diseases in refugees and asylum seekers—Current status and going forward. *Public Health Rev.* **2017**, *38*, 22. [CrossRef]

25. Pohl, C.; Mack, I.; Schmitz, T.; Ritz, N. The spectrum of care for pediatric refugees and asylum seekers at a tertiary health care facility in Switzerland in 2015. *Eur. J. Pediatr.* **2017**, *176*, 1681–1687. [CrossRef]
26. Kampouras, A.; Tzikos, G.; Partsanakis, E.; Roukas, K.; Tsiamitros, S.; Deligeorgakis, D.; Chorafa, E.; Schoina, M.; Iosifidis, E. Child morbidity and disease burden in refugee camps in mainland Greece. *Children* **2019**, *6*, 46. [CrossRef]
27. Staat, M.A. Infectious diseases in refugee and internationally adopted children. In *Principles and Practice of Pediatric Infectious Diseases*, 5th ed.; Long, S.S., Prober, C.G., Fisher, M., Eds.; Elsevier: Philadelphia, PA, USA, 2018; pp. 32–36.
28. American Academy of Pediatrics Council on Community Pediatrics. Providing care for immigrant, migrant, and border children. *Pediatrics* **2013**, *131*, e2028–e2034. [CrossRef]
29. Mitchell, T.; Weinberg, M.; Posey, D.L.; Cetron, M. Immigrant and refugee health: A Centers for Disease Control and Prevention perspective on protecting the health and health security of individuals and communities during planned migration. *Pediatr. Clin. N. Am.* **2019**, *66*, 549–560. [CrossRef]
30. Barnett, E.D. Infectious disease screening for refugees resettled in the United States. *Clin. Infect. Dis.* **2004**, *39*, 833–841. [CrossRef] [PubMed]
31. Centers for Disease Control and Prevention. Guidelines for the U.S. Domestic Medical Examination for Newly Arriving Refugees. Available online: http://www.cdc.gov/immigrantrefugeehealth/guidelines/general-guidelines.html (accessed on 20 July 2019).
32. Centers for Disease Control and Prevention. International Adoption: Health Guidance and Immigration Process for Parents: Finding a Medical Provider in the United States. Available online: http://cdc.gov/immigrantrefugeehealth/adoption/finding-doctor.html (accessed on 20 July 2019).
33. Centers for Disease Control and Prevention. Medical Examination of Immigrants and Refugees. Available online: https://www.cdc.gov/immigrantrefugeehealth/exams/medical-examination.html (accessed on 20 July 2019).
34. Centers for Disease Control and Prevention. Immigrant and Refugee Health. Available online: https://www.cdc.gov/immigrantrefugeehealth/guidelines/refugee-guidelines.html (accessed on 20 July 2019).
35. Centers for Disease Control and Prevention. Technical Instructions for Civil Surgeons. Available online: https://www.cdc.gov/immigrantrefugeehealth/exams/ti/civil/technical-instructions-civil-surgeons.html. (accessed on 26 November 2019).
36. American Academy of Pediatrics. Immigrant Child Health Toolkit. Available online: https://www.aap.org/en-us/advocacy-and-policy/aap-health-initiatives/Immigrant-Child-Health-Toolkit/Pages/Immigrant-Child-Health-Toolkit.aspx (accessed on 20 July 2019).
37. UNAIDS. Fact Sheet—Global AIDS Update 2019. Available online: https://www.unaids.org/sites/default/files/media_asset/UNAIDS_FactSheet_en.pdf (accessed on 20 July 2019).
38. Del Amo, J.; Likatavicius, G.; Perez-Cachafeiro, S.; Hernando, V.; Gonzalez, C.; Jarrin, I.; Noori, T.; Hamers, F.F.; Bolumar, F. The epidemiology of HIV and AIDS reports in migrants in the 27 European Union countries, Norway and Iceland: 1999–2006. *Eur. J. Public Health* **2011**, *21*, 620–626. [CrossRef] [PubMed]
39. McCarthy, A.E.; Weld, L.H.; Barnett, E.D.; So, H.; Coyle, C.; Greenaway, C.; Stauffer, W.; Leder, K.; Lopez-Velez, R.; Gautret, P.; et al. Spectrum of illness in international migrants seen at GeoSentinel clinics in 1997–2009, part 2: Migrants resettled internationally and evaluated for specific health concerns. GeoSentinel Surveillance Network. *Clin. Infect. Dis.* **2013**, *56*, 925–933. [CrossRef] [PubMed]
40. Kortas, A.Z.; Polenz, J.; von Hayek, J.; Rudiger, S.; Rottbauer, W.; Storr, U.; Wibmer, T. Screening for infectious diseases among asylum seekers newly arrived in Germany in 2015: A systematic single-centre analysis. *Public Health* **2017**, *153*, 1–8. [CrossRef]
41. Redditt, V.J.; Janakiram, P.; Graziano, D.; Rashid, M. Health status of newly arrived refugees in Toronto, Ont: Part 1: Infectious diseases. *Can. Fam. Physician* **2015**, *1*, e303–e309.
42. Centers for Disease Control and Prevention. Screening for HIV Infection During the Refugee Domestic Medical Examination. Available online: https://www.cdc.gov/immigrantrefugeehealth/guidelines/domestic/screening-hiv-infection-domestic.html (accessed on 20 July 2019).
43. Panel on Opportunistic Infections in HIV-Exposed and HIV-Infected Children. Guidelines for the Prevention and Treatment of Opportunistic Infections among HIV-Exposed and HIV-infected Children. Available online: https://aidsinfo.nih.gov/contentfiles/lvguidelines/oi_guidelines_pediatrics.pdf (accessed on 20 July 2019).

44. Odone, A.; Tillman, T.; Sandgreen, A.; Williams, G.; Rechel, B.; Ingleby, D.; Noori, T.; Mladovsky, P.; McKee, M. Tuberculosis among migrant populations in the European Union and the European economic area. *Eur. J. Public Health* **2014**, *18*, 405–412. [CrossRef]
45. Marras, T.K.; Wilson, J.; Wang, E.E.; Avendano, M.; Yang, J.W. Tuberculosis among Tibetan refugee claimants in Toronto: 1998 to 2000. *Chest* **2003**, *124*, 915–921. [CrossRef]
46. Ritz, N.; Curtis, N. Novel concepts in the epidemiology, diagnosis and prevention of childhood tuberculosis. *Swiss Med. Wkly.* **2014**, *144*, w14000. [CrossRef]
47. Jenkins, H.E.; Yuen, C.M.; Rodriguez, C.A.; Nathavitharana, R.R.; McLaughlin, M.M.; Donald, P.; Marais, B.J.; Becerra, M.C. Mortality in children diagnosed with tuberculosis: A systematic review and meta-analysis. *Lancet Infect. Dis.* **2017**, *17*, 285–295. [CrossRef]
48. Mueller-Hermelink, M.; Kobbe, R.; Methling, B.; Rau, C.; Schulze-Sturm, U.; Auer, I.; Ahrens, F.; Brinkmann, F. Universal screening for latent and active tuberculosis (TB) in asylum seeking childn, Bochum and Hamburg, Germany, September 2015 to November 2016. *Eur. Surveill.* **2018**, *23*. [CrossRef]
49. Oesch Nemeth, G.; Nemeth, J.; Altpeter, E.; Ritz, N. Epidemiology of childhood tuberculosis in Switzerland between 1996 and 2011. *Eur. J. Pediatr.* **2014**, *173*, 457–462. [CrossRef] [PubMed]
50. Aldridge, R.W.; Zenner, D.; White, P.J.; Williamson, E.J.; Muzyamba, M.C.; Dhavan, P.; Mosca, D.; Thomas, H.L.; Lalor, M.K.; Abubakar, I.; et al. Tuberculosis in migrants moving from high incidence to low-incidence countries: A population-based cohort study of 519 955 migrants screened before entry to England, Wales, and Northern Ireland. *Lancet* **2016**, *388*, 2510–2518. [CrossRef]
51. Liu, Y.; Weinberg, M.S.; Ortega, L.S.; Painter, J.A.; Maloney, S.A. Overseas screening for tuberculosis in U.S.-bound immigrants and refugees. *N. Engl. J. Med.* **2009**, *360*, 2406–2415. [CrossRef] [PubMed]
52. Yun, K.; Matheson, J.; Payton, C.; Scott, K.C.; Stone, B.L.; Song, L.; Stauffer, W.M.; Urban, K.; Young, J.; Mamo, B. Health profiles of newly arrived refugee children in the United States, 2006–2012. *Am. J. Public Health* **2016**, *106*, 128–135. [CrossRef] [PubMed]
53. Marquardt, L.; Kramer, A.; Fischer, F.; Prufer-Kramer, L. Health status and disease burden of unaccompanied asylum seeking adolescents in Bielefeld, Germany: Cross-sectional pilot study. *Trop. Med. Int. Health* **2016**, *21*, 210–218. [CrossRef] [PubMed]
54. Centers for Disease Control and Prevention. Tuberculosis Technical Instructions for Panel Physicians. Available online: https://www.cdc.gov/immigrantrefugeehealth/exams/ti/panel/tuberculosis-panel-technical-instructions.html (accessed on 31 July 2019).
55. Pai, M.; Zwerling, A.; Menzies, D. Systematic review: T-cell based assays for the diagnosis of latent tuberculosis infection: An update. *Ann. Intern. Med.* **2008**, *149*, 177–184. [CrossRef]
56. Starke, J.R. American Academy of Pediatrics, Committee on Infectious Diseases, Technical report: Interferon-gamma-release assay for diagnosis of tuberculous infection and disease in children. *Pediatrics* **2014**, *134*, e1763–e1773. [CrossRef]
57. European Centre for Disease Prevention and Control. *Cost Effectiveness Analysis of Programmatic Screening Strategies for Latent Tuberculosis Infection in the EU/EEA*; ECDC, Stockholm: Solna Municipality, Sweden, 2018.
58. Usemann, J.; Ledergerber, M.; Fink, G.; Ritz, N. Cost effectiveness of tuberculosis screening for migrant children in a low-incidence country. *Int. J. Tuberc. Lung Dis.* **2019**, *23*, 579–586. [CrossRef]
59. Zammarchi, L.; Casadei, G.; Strohmeyer, M.; Bartalesi, F.; Liendo, C.; Matteelli, A.; Bonati, M.; Gotuzzo, E.; Bartoloni, A.; COHEMI Project Study Group. A scoping review of cost-effectiveness of screening and treatment for latent tuberculosis infection in migrants from high-incidence countries. *BMC Health Serv. Res.* **2015**, *15*, 412. [CrossRef]
60. Nyangoma, E.N.; Olson, C.K.; Painter, J.A.; Posey, D.L.; Stauffer, W.M.; Naughton, M.; Zhou, W.; Kamb, M.; Benoit, S.R. Syphilis among U.S.-bound refugees, 2009–2013. *J. Immigr. Minor. Health* **2017**, *19*, 835–842. [CrossRef]
61. Workowski, K.A.; Bolan, G.A. Centers for Disease Control and Prevention. Sexually transmitted diseases treatment guidelines, 2015. *MMWR Recomm. Rep.* **2015**, *64*, 1–137. [PubMed]
62. Mellou, K.; Chrisostomou, A.; Sideroglou, T.; Georgakopoulou, T.; Kyritsi, M.; Hadjichristodoulou, C.; Tsiodras, S. Hepatitis A among refugees, asylum seekers and migrants living in hosting facilities, Greece, April to December 2016. *Eur. Surveill.* **2017**, *22*, 30448. [CrossRef] [PubMed]

63. Michaelis, K.; Wenzel, J.J.; Stark, K.; Faber, M. Hepatitis A virus infections and outbreaks in asylum seekers arriving to Germany, September 2015 to March 2016. *Emerg. Microbes Infect.* **2017**, *6*, e26. [CrossRef] [PubMed]
64. Jablonka, A.; Solbach, P.; Wöbse, M.; Manns, M.P.; Schmidt, R.E.; Wedemeyer, H.; Cornberg, M.; Behrens, G.M.N.; Hardtke, S. Seroprevalence of antibodies and antigens against hepatitis A-E viruses in refugees and asylum seekers in Germany in 2015. *Eur. J. Gastroenterol. Hepatol.* **2017**, *29*, 939–945. [CrossRef]
65. Hutin, Y.; Nasrullah, M.; Easterbrook, P.; Nguimfack, B.D.; Burrone, E.; Averhoff, F.; Bulterys, M. Access to treatment for hepatitis B virus infection—Worldwide 2016. *MMWR Morb. Mortal. Wkly. Rep.* **2018**, *67*, 773–777. [CrossRef] [PubMed]
66. World Health Organization (WHO). *Global Hepatitis Report, 2017*; World Health Organization: Geneva, Switzerland, 2017.
67. Indolfi, G.; Easterbrook, P.; Dusheiko, G.; Siberry, G.; Chang, M.H.; Bulterys, T.C.; Chan, P.L.; El-Sayed, M.H.; Giaquinto, C.; Jonas, M.M.; et al. Hepatitis B virus infection in children and adolescents. *Lancet Gastroenterol. Hepatol.* **2019**, *4*, 466–476. [CrossRef]
68. Serre Delcor, N.; Maruri, B.T.; Arandes, A.S.; Guiu, I.C.; Essadik, H.O.; Soley, M.E.; Romero, I.M.; Ascaso, C. Infectious diseases in Sub-Saharan immigrants to Spain. *Am. J. Trop. Med. Hyg.* **2016**, *94*, 750–756. [CrossRef]
69. Coppola, N.; Alessio, L.; Gualdieri, L.; Pisaturo, M.; Sagnelli, C.; Minichini, C.; Di Caprio, G.; Starace, M.; Onorato, L.; Signoriello, G.; et al. Hepatitis B virus infection in undocumented immigrants and refugees in southern Italy: Demographic, virological, and clinical features. *Infect. Dis. Poverty* **2017**, *6*, 33. [CrossRef]
70. Cai, W.; Poethko-Muller, C.; Hamouda, O.; Radun, D. Hepatitis B virus infections among children and adolescents in Germany: Migration background as a risk factor in a low seroprevalence population. *Pediatr. Infect. Dis. J.* **2011**, *30*, 19–24. [CrossRef]
71. Edmunds, W.J.; Medley, G.F.; Nokes, D.J.; Hall, A.J.; Whittle, H.C. The influence of age on the development of the hepatitis B carrier state. *Proc. Biol. Sci.* **1993**, *253*, 197–201.
72. Centers for Disease Control and Prevention. A comprehensive immunization strategy to eliminate Hepatitis B virus infection in the Unites States. Recommendations of the Advisory Committee on Immunization Practices (ACIP). Part II: Immunization of adults. *MMWR Recomm. Rep.* **2005**, *55*, 1–33.
73. Hahne, S.J.; Veldhuijzen, I.K.; Wiessing, L.; Lim, T.A.; Salminen, M.; Laar, M. Infection with hepatitis B and C virus in Europe: A systematic review of prevalence and cost-effectiveness of screening. *BMC Infect. Dis.* **2013**, *13*, 181. [CrossRef] [PubMed]
74. Jazwa, A.; Coleman, M.S.; Gazmararian, J.; Wingate, L.T.; Maskery, B.; Mitchell, T.; Weinberg, M. Cost-benefit comparison of two proposed overseas programs for reducing chronic hepatitis infection among refugees: Is screening essential. *Vaccine* **2015**, *33*, 1393–1399. [CrossRef] [PubMed]
75. Indolfi, G.; Easterbrook, P.; Dusheiko, G.; El-Sayed, M.H.; Jonas, M.M.; Thorne, C.; Bulterys, M.; Siberry, G.; Walsh, N.; Chang, M.H.; et al. Hepatitis C virus infection in children and adolescents. *Lancet Gastroenterol. Hepatol.* **2019**, *4*, 477–487. [CrossRef]
76. Ng, E.; Sanmartin, C.; Elien-Massenat, D.; Manuel, D.G. Vaccine-preventable disease-related hospitalization among immigrants and refugees to Canada: Study of linked population-based databases. *Vaccine* **2016**, *34*, 4437–4442. [CrossRef]
77. Charania, N.A.; Paynter, J.; Lee, A.C.; Watson, D.G.; Turner, N.M. Vaccine-preventable disease-associated hospitalisations among migrant and non-migrant children in New Zealand. *J. Immigr. Minor. Health* **2019**, 1–9. [CrossRef]
78. Charania, N.A.; Gaze, N.; Kung, J.Y.; Brooks, S. Vaccine-preventable diseases and immunisation coverage among migrants and non-migrants worldwide: A scoping review of published literature, 2006 to 2016. *Vaccine* **2019**, *37*, 2661–2669. [CrossRef]
79. Carrico, R.M.; Goss, L.; Wiemken, T.L.; Bosson, R.S.; Peyrani, P.; Mattingly, W.A.; Pauly, A.; Ford, R.A.; Kotey, S.; Ramirez, J.A. Infection prevention and control and the refugee population: Experiences from the University of Louisville Global Health Center. *Am. J. Infect. Control* **2017**, *45*, 673–676. [CrossRef]
80. Luman, E.T.; McCauley, M.M.; Stokley, S.; Chu, S.Y.; Pickering, L.K. Timeliness of childhood immunizations. *Pediatrics* **2002**, *110*, 935–939. [CrossRef]

81. Ravensbergen, S.J.; Nellums, L.B.; Hargreaves, S.; Stienstra, Y.; Friedland, J.S. ESGITM working group on vaccination in migrants. national approaches to the vaccination of recently arrived migrants in Europe: A comparative policy analysis across 32 European countries. *Travel. Med. Infect. Dis.* **2019**, *27*, 33–38. [CrossRef]
82. Hargreaves, S.; Nellums, L.B.; Ravensbergen, S.J.; Friedland, J.S.; Stienstra, Y.; On Behalf of the Esgitm Working Group on Vaccination in Migrants. Divergent approaches in the vaccination of recently arrived migrants to Europe: A survey of national experts from 32 countries, 2017. *Eur. Surveill.* **2018**, *23*. [CrossRef] [PubMed]
83. Hagstam, P.; Böttiger, B.; Winqvist, N. Measles and rubella seroimmunity in newly arrived adult immigrants in Sweden. *Infect. Dis. (Lond.)* **2019**, *51*, 122–130. [CrossRef] [PubMed]
84. Hall, V.; Banerjee, E.; Kenyon, C.; Strain, A.; Griffith, J.; Como-Sabetti, K.; Heath, J.; Bahta, L.; Martin, K.; McMahon, M.; et al. Measles outbreak—Minnesota, April–May, 2017. *MMWR Morb. Mortal. Wkly. Rep.* **2017**, *66*, 713–717. [CrossRef]
85. Nysse, L.J.; Pinsky, N.A.; Bratberg, J.P.; Babar-Weber, A.Y.; Samuel, T.T.; Krych, E.H.; Ziegler, A.W.; Jimale, M.A.; Vierkant, R.A.; Jacobson, R.M.; et al. Seroprevalence of antibody to varicella among Somali refugees. *Mayo Clin. Proc.* **2007**, *82*, 175–180. [CrossRef]
86. Leeds, M.; Muscoplat, M.H. Timeliness of receipt of early childhood vaccinations among children of immigrants—Minnesota, 2016. *MMWR Morb. Mortal. Wkly. Rep.* **2017**, *66*, 1125–1129. [CrossRef] [PubMed]
87. Wolff, E.R.; Madlon-Kay, D.J. Childhood vaccine beliefs reported by Somali and non-Somali parents. *J. Am. Board Fam. Med.* **2014**, *27*, 458–464. [CrossRef]
88. Kamadjeu, R.; Mahamud, A.; Webeck, J.; Baranyikwa, M.T.; Chatterjee, A.; Bile, Y.N.; Birungi, J.; Mbaeyi, C.; Mulugeta, A. Polio outbreak investigation and response in Somalia, 2013. *J. Infect. Dis.* **2014**, *210* (Suppl. 1), S181–S186. [CrossRef]
89. Walker, A.T.; Sodha, S.; Warren, W.C.; Sergon, K.; Kiptoon, S.; Ogange, J.; Ahmeda, A.H.; Eshetu, M.; Corkum, M.; Pillai, S. Forewarning of poliovirus outbreaks in the Horn of Africa: An assessment of acute flaccid paralysis surveillance and routine immunization systems in Kenya. *J. Infect. Dis.* **2014**, *210* (Suppl. 1), S85–S90. [CrossRef]
90. Ozaras, R.; Leblebicioglu, H.; Sunbul, M.; Tabak, F.; Balkan, I.I.; Yemisen, M.; Sencan, I.; Ozturk, R. The Syrian conflict and infectious diseases. *Expert Rev. Anti-Infect. Ther.* **2016**, *14*, 547–555. [CrossRef]
91. Heudtlass, P.; Speybroeck, N.; Guha-Sapir, D. Excess mortality in refugees, internally displaced persons and resident populations in complex humanitarian emergencies (1998–2012)—Insights from operational data. *Confl. Health* **2016**, *10*, 15. [CrossRef]
92. Weatherhead, J.E.; Hotez, P.J. Worm infection in children. *Pediatr. Rev.* **2015**, *36*, 341–354. [CrossRef] [PubMed]
93. Swanson, S.J.; Phares, C.R.; Mamo, B.; Smith, K.E.; Cetron, M.S.; Stauffer, W.M. Albendazole therapy and enteric parasites in United States-bound refugees. *N. Engl. J. Med.* **2012**, *366*, 1498–1507. [CrossRef]
94. Heudorf, U.; Karathana, M.; Krackhardt, B.; Huber, M.; Raupp, P.; Zinn, C. Surveillance for parasites in unaccompanied minor refugees migrating to Germany in 2015. *GMS Hyg. Infect. Control* **2016**, *11*, Doc05. [PubMed]
95. Posey, D.L.; Blackburn, B.G.; Weinberg, M.; Flagg, E.W.; Ortega, L.; Wilson, M.; Secor, W.E.; Sanders-Lewis, K.; Won, K.; Maguire, J.H. High prevalence and presumptive treatment of schistosomiasis and strongyloidiasis among African refugees. *Clin. Infect. Dis.* **2007**, *45*, 1310–1315. [CrossRef] [PubMed]
96. Marchese, V.; Beltrame, A.; Angheben, A.; Monteiro, G.B.; Giorli, G.; Perandin, F.; Buonfrate, D.; Bisoffi, Z. Schistosomiasis in immigrants, refugees and travelers in an Italian referral centre for tropical diseases. *Infect. Dis. Poverty* **2018**, *7*, 55. [CrossRef]
97. Poddighe, D.; Castelli, L.; Pulcrano, G.; Grosini, A.; Balzaretti, M.; Spadaro, S.; Bruni, P. Urinary Schistosomiasis in an adolescent refugee from Africa: an uncommon cause of Hematuria and an emerging infectious disease in Europe. *J. Immigr. Minor. Health.* **2016**, *18*, 1237–1240. [CrossRef] [PubMed]
98. Theuring, S.; Friedrich-Janicke, B.; Portner, K.; Trebesch, I.; Durst, A.; Dieckmann, S.; Steiner, F.; Harms, G.; Mockenhaupt, F.P. Screening for infectious diseases among unaccompanied minor refugees in Berlin, 2014–2015. *Eur. J. Epidemiol.* **2016**, *31*, 707–710. [CrossRef] [PubMed]
99. Greaves, D.; Coggle, S.; Pollard, C.; Aliyu, S.H.; Moore, E.M. Strongyloides stercoralis infection. *BMJ* **2013**, *347*, f4610. [CrossRef]

100. Buonfrate, D.; Requena-Mendez, A.; Angheben, A.; Munoz, J.; Gobbi, F.; Van Den Ende, J.; Bisoffi, Z. Severe strongyloidiasis: A systematic review of case reports. *BMC Infect. Dis.* **2013**, *13*, 78. [CrossRef]
101. Chernet, A.; Kling, K.; Sydow, V.; Kuenzli, E.; Hatz, C.; Utzinger, J.; van Lieshout, L.; Marti, H.; Nickel, B.; Labhardt, N.D.; et al. Accuracy of diagnostic tests for Schistosoma mansoni infection in asymptomatic Eritrean refugees: Serology and POC-CCA against stool microscopy. *Clin. Infect. Dis.* **2017**, *65*, 568–574. [CrossRef]
102. Puthiyakunnon, S.; Boddu, S.; Li, Y.; Zhou, X.; Wang, C.; Li, J.; Chen, X. Strongyloidiasis—An insight into its global prevalence and management. *PLoS. Negl. Trop. Dis.* **2014**, *8*, e3018. [CrossRef] [PubMed]
103. Pérez-Molina, J.A.; Molina, I. Chagas disease. *Lancet* **2018**, *391*, 82–94. [CrossRef]
104. World Health Organization. World Malaria Report 2016. Available online: https://www.who.int/malaria/publications/world-malaria-report2016/report/en/ (accessed on 21 July 2019).
105. Crawley, J.; Chu, C.; Mtove, G.; Nosten, F. Malaria in children. *Lancet* **2010**, *375*, 1468–1481. [CrossRef]
106. Di Meco, E.; Di Napoli, A.; Amato, L.M.; Fortino, A.; Costanzo, G.; Rossi, A.; Mirisola, C.; Petrelli, A. Infectious and dermatological diseases among arriving migrants on the Italian coasts. *Eur. J. Public. Health.* **2018**, *28*, 910–916. [CrossRef] [PubMed]
107. Greenaway, C.; Castelli, F. Infectious diseases at different stages of migration: An expert review. *J. Travel Med.* **2019**, *26*, taz007. [CrossRef] [PubMed]
108. Williams, G.A.; Bacci, S.; Shadwick, R.; Tillmann, T.; Rechel, B.; Noori, T.; Suk, J.E.; Odone, A.; Ingleby, J.D.; Mladovsky, P.; et al. Measles among migrants in the European Union and the European Economic Area. *Scand. J. Public Health* **2016**, *44*, 6–13. [CrossRef]
109. Hoch, M.; Wieser, A.; Loscher, T.; Margos, G.; Purner, F.; Zuhl, J.; Seilmaier, M.; Balzer, L.; Guggemos, W.; Rack-Hoch, A.; et al. Louse-borne relapsing fever (*Borrelia recurrentis*) diagnosed in 15 refugees from Northeast Africa: Epidemiology and preventive control measures, Bavaria, Germany, July to October 2015. *Euro. Surveill.* **2015**, *20*. [CrossRef]
110. Centers for Disease Control and Prevention. General recommendations on immunization: Recommendations of the Advisory Committee on Immunization Practices (ACIP). *MMWR Recomm. Rep.* **2011**, *60*, 1–64.
111. Pickering, L.K.; Baker, C.J.; Freed, G.L.; Gall, S.A.; Grogg, S.E.; Poland, G.A.; Rodewald, L.E.; Schaffner, W.; Stinchfield, P.; Tan, L.; et al. Immunization programs for infants, children, adolescents, and adults: Clinical practice guidelines by the Infectious Diseases Society of America. *Clin. Infect. Dis.* **2009**, *49*, 817–840. [CrossRef]
112. American Academy of Pediatrics. Immunization in special clinical circumstances: Refugees and immigrants. In *Red Book 2015: Report of the Committee on Infectious Diseases*, 30th ed.; Kimberlin, D.W., Brady, M.T., Jackson, M.A., Long, S.S., Eds.; American Academy of Pediatrics: Elk Grove Village, IL, USA, 2015.
113. Figueira, M.D.; Christiansen, D.; Barnett, E.D. Cost-effectiveness of sero-testing compared with universal immunization for varicella in refugee children from 6 geographic regions. *J. Travel Med.* **2003**, *10*, 203–213. [CrossRef]
114. Zimmerman, C.; Kiss, L.; Hossain, M. Migration and health: A framework for 21st century policy-making. *PLoS Med.* **2011**, *8*, e1001034. [CrossRef] [PubMed]
115. Pottie, K.; Greenaway, C.; Feightner, J.; Welch, V.; Swinkels, H.; Rashid, M.; Narasiah, L.; Kirmayer, L.J.; Uffing, E.; MacDonald, N.E.; et al. Evidence-based clinical guidelines for immigrants and refugees. *CMAJ* **2011**, *183*, E824–E925. [CrossRef] [PubMed]
116. Maskery, B.; Coleman, M.S.; Weinberg, M.; Zhou, W.; Rotz, L.; Klosovsky, A.; Cantey, P.T.; Fox, L.M.; Cetron, M.S.; Stauffer, W.M. Economic analysis of the impact of overseas and domestic treatment and screening options for intestinal helminth infection among US-bound refugees from Asia. *PLoS. Negl. Trop. Dis.* **2016**, *10*, e0004910. [CrossRef]
117. Migrant Health Assessment Sub-Committee of HPSC Scientific Advisory Committee. Infectious Disease Assessment for Migrants Toolkit. Health Protection Surveillance Centre. 2015. Available online: http://www.hpsc.ie/A-Z/SpecificPopulations/Migrants/ (accessed on 24 September 2016).

118. Chaves, N.J.; Paxton, G.; Biggs, B.A.; Thambiran, A.; Smith, M.; Williams, J.; Gardiner, J.; Davis, J.S.; On Behalf of the Australasian Society for Infectious Diseases and Refugee Health Network of Australia Guidelines Writing Group. Recommendations for comprehensive post-arrival health assessment for people from refugee-like backgrounds. In *Australasian Society for Infectious Diseases and Refugee Health Network of Australia*, 2nd ed.; Australasian Society for Infectious Diseases Inc: Surry Hills, Australia, 2016. Available online: https://www.asid.net.au/documents/item/1225 (accessed on 15 March 2017).
119. Bradby, H.; Humphris, R.; Newall, D.; Philimore, J. *Public Health Aspects of Migrant Health A Review of the Evidence on Health Status for Refugees and Asylum Seekers in the European Region*; Health Evidence Network Synthesis Report No.: 44; World Health Organization: Geneva, Switzerland, 2015. Available online: http://www.euro.who.int/__data/assets/pdf_file/0004/289246/WHO-HEN-Report-A5-2-Refugees_FINAL.pdf (accessed on 26 November 2019).
120. Seedat, F.; Hargreaves, S.; Nellums, L.B.; Ouyang, J.; Brown, M.; Friedland, J.S. How effective are approaches to migrant screening for infectious diseases in Europe? A systematic review. *Lancet Infect. Dis.* **2018**, *18*, e259–e271. [CrossRef]
121. European Centre for Disease Prevention and Control. Guidance on Tuberculosis Control in Vulnerable and Hard-to-Reach Populations. 2016. Available online: http://ecdc.europa.eu/en/publications/_layouts/forms/Publication_DispForm.aspx?List=4f55ad51-4aed-4d32-b960-af70113dbb90&ID=1451 (accessed on 19 July 2019).
122. United Nations. *Convention on the Rights of the Child*; United Nations: Geneva, Switzerland, 1989.
123. Pottie, K.; Hui, C.; Rahman, P.; Ingleby, D.; Akl, E.A.; Russell, G.; Ling, L.; Wickramage, K.; Mosca, D.; Brindis, C.D. Building responsive health systems to help communities affected by migration: an international Delphi consensus. *Int. J. Environ. Res. Public Health* **2017**, *14*, 20144. [CrossRef] [PubMed]
124. Seiber, E.E. Which states enroll their Medicaid eligible, citizen children with immigrant parents. *Health Serv. Res.* **2013**, *48*, 519–538. [CrossRef]
125. Hui, C.; Dunn, J.; Morton, R.; Staub, L.; Tran, A.; Hargreaves, S. Interventions to improve vaccination uptake and Cost Effectiveness of vaccination strategies in newly arrived migrants in the EU/EEA: A systematic review. *Int. J. Environ. Res. Public Health* **2018**, *15*, 2065. [CrossRef]
126. Pezzi, C.; McCulloch, A.; Joo, H.; Cochran, J.; Smock, L.; Frerich, E.; Mamo, B.; Urban, K.; Hughes, S.; Payton, C.; et al. Vaccine delivery to newly arrived refugees and estimated costs in selected U.S. clinics, 2015. *Vaccine* **2018**, *36*, 2902–2909. [CrossRef]
127. Morales, M.; Nnadi, C.D.; Tangermann, R.H.; Wassilak, S.G. Notes from the field: Circulating vaccine-derived poliovirus outbreaks—Five countries, 2014–2015. *MMWR Morb. Mortal. Wkly. Rep.* **2016**, *65*, 128–129. [CrossRef]
128. Nnadi, C.; Etsano, A.; Uba, B.; Ohuabunwo, C.; Melton, M.; Wa Nganda, G.; Esapa, L.; Bolu, O.; Mahoney, F.; Vertefeuille, J.; et al. Approaches to vaccination among populations in areas of conflict. *J. Infect. Dis.* **2017**, *216* (Suppl. 1), S368–S372. [CrossRef]
129. Gunst, M.; Jarman, K.; Yarwood, V.; Rokadiya, S.; Capsaskis, L.; Orcutt, M.; Abbara, A. Healthcare access for refugees in Greece: Challenges and opportunities. *Health Policy* **2019**, *123*, 818–824. [CrossRef] [PubMed]
130. International Society for Social Pediatrics and Child Health (ISSOP). ISSOP position statement on migrant child health. *Child Care Health Dev.* **2018**, *44*, 161–170. [CrossRef] [PubMed]
131. Zwi, K.; Morton, N.; Woodland, L.; Mallitt, K.A.; Palasanthiran, P. Screening and primary care access for newly arrived paediatric refugees in regional Australia: A 5 year cross-sectional analysis (2007-12). *J. Trop. Pediatr.* **2017**, *63*, 109–117. [CrossRef]
132. Woodland, L.; Burgner, D.; Paxton, B.A.; Zwi, K. Health service delivery for newly arrived refugee children: A framework for good practice. *J. Paediatr. Child Health.* **2010**, *46*, 560–567. [CrossRef]
133. Enriquez, L.E. Multigenerational punishment: Shared experiences of undocumented immigration status within mixed-status families. *J. Marriage Fam.* **2015**, *77*, 939–953. [CrossRef]
134. US Department of Homeland Security. *United States Border Patrol Southwest Family Unit and Unaccompanied Alien Children Apprehensions Fiscal Year 2016*; Customs and Border Protection: Washington, DC, USA, 2016. Available online: https://www.cbp.gov/newsroom/stats/southwest-border-unaccompanied-children/fy-2016 (accessed on 21 December 2016).
135. Linton, J.M.; Nagda, J.; Falusi, O.O. Advocating for immigration policies that promote children's health. *Pediatr. Clin. N. Am.* **2019**, *66*, 619–640. [CrossRef]

136. Linton, J.M.; Griffin, M.; Shapiro, A.J.; Council on Community Pediatrics. Detention of immigrant children. *Pediatrics* **2017**, *139*, e20170483. [CrossRef]
137. Eskenazi, B.; Fahey, C.A.; Kogut, K.; Gunier, R.; Torres, J.; Gonzales, N.A.; Holland, N.; Deardorff, J. Association of perceived immigration policy vulnerability with mental and physical health among US-born Latino adolescents in California. *JAMA Pediatr.* **2019**, *173*. [CrossRef]
138. Dawson-Hahn, E.; Chazaro, A. Mitigating the health consequences for youth in families affected by immigration policy changes: Opportunities for health care professionals and health systems. *JAMA Pediatr.* **2019**, *173*, 721–723. [CrossRef]

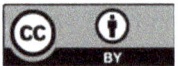

© 2019 by the author. Licensee MDPI, Basel, Switzerland. This article is an open access article distributed under the terms and conditions of the Creative Commons Attribution (CC BY) license (http://creativecommons.org/licenses/by/4.0/).

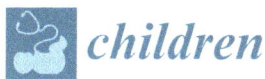

Review

The Importance of Oral Health in Immigrant and Refugee Children

Eileen Crespo

Department of Pediatrics, Hennepin County Medical Center, Minneapolis, MN 55415, USA; eileen.crespo@hcmed.org

Received: 26 June 2019; Accepted: 3 September 2019; Published: 9 September 2019

Abstract: According to the Migration Policy Institute, 2017 data revealed that a historic high 44.5 million people living in the United States (US) were foreign-born (Zong, J., et.al., 2019), more than double the number from 1990 (U.S. Immigrant Population and Share over Time. 1850-Present, 2019). Since the creation of the Refugee Resettlement Program in 1980, refugee families have settled in the US more than in any other country in the world (Radford, J., 2019). In 2018, for the first time, Canada overtook the US in numbers of refugees accepted (Zong, J., et. al., 2019). Foreign-born people now account for 13.7% of the total US population (Zong, J., et. al., 2019). Further, a quarter of children in the United States currently live in households with at least one foreign-born parent (America's Children in Brief: Key National Indicators of Well-Being, 2018). These population shifts are important to note because immigrant and refugee families bring cultural influences and health experiences from their home countries which can greatly affect the overall health and well-being of children. For these new arrivals, oral health is often a significant health issue. The severity of dental disease varies with country of origin as well as cultural beliefs that can hinder access to care even once it is available to them (Obeng, C.S. Culture and dental health among African immigrant school-aged children in the United States, 200; Tiwari, T.; Albino, J. Acculturation and Pediatric Minority Oral Health Interventions, 2017). As pediatricians and primary care providers, we should acknowledge that oral health is important and impacts overall health. Healthcare providers should be able to recognize oral health problems, make appropriate referrals, and effectively communicate with families to address knowledge gaps in high-risk communities.

Keywords: oral health; immigrant and refugee children; culturally responsive care; acculturation

1. Background

Latinos are the largest ethnic group in the US and are projected to be the dominant minority group by 2044 [1]. Mexico accounts for the largest group of immigrants in the US, responsible for 25% of all immigrants [2]. However, there has been a shift noted since 2010 with larger numbers of immigrants coming from countries in South and East Asia such as India and China [2]. The number of immigrants of Asian origin is growing so quickly that they are expected to surpass Latinos to become the largest immigrant group in the United States by 2055 [2]. Additionally, because foreign-born women tend to have higher fertility rates [3], it is projected that by 2020, more than half of the children in the United States will have parents who are foreign-born [4].

According to 2015–2016 data from the National Health and Nutrition Examination Survey (NHANES), Hispanic children have the highest prevalence of dental caries of children aged 2–19 years in the US [5]. The rates for Hispanic children were higher than for all other groups surveyed at 57.1% and significantly higher than for non-Hispanic white children [5]. It Is important to note that as the largest immigrant group in the US that also suffers from the highest prevalence of dental disease, children of Hispanic immigrants may benefit from enhanced oral health screening and appropriate referral in the primary care setting.

Refugees coming to the US are another group at high risk of caries. A recent study showed a 64% higher caries risk rates in refugee children from Asia compared with African refugee children [6]. The refugee children from Asia also had more urgent unmet dental needs than refugees from Africa, 46.1% vs. 30%, respectively [6]. According to 2018 Pew Research data, the majority of refugees to the US are arriving from Africa, Eastern Europe, the Middle East, and Asia [4]. Since the United States government started the Refugee Resettlement Program, three million refugees have come to the US. While the total number of refugees is lower than that of immigrants, refugees can be at higher risk for poor oral health due to multiple factors. Some of these factors, which are described in detail, include home country, cultural influences including diet and health beliefs, as well as time spent in refugee camps where cariogenic foods have historically been available [7].

2. Role of Country of Origin

Country of origin has an impact on the rate of dental caries because access to dental care, traditional diet, access to refined sugars, exposure to fluoride, and personal hygiene practices all affect the risk of developing caries. Cote and colleagues found marked differences in groups of refugee children screened for dental caries upon arrival in the US. In the population studied, refugee children from East African countries had surprisingly low rates of caries, even lower than African-American children from the US, despite many of them having never had a dental visit nor practiced routine dental hygiene [8]. Refugee children from Eastern European countries had the highest rates of caries experience in this study. Refugee children from Eastern European countries were 5.6 times more likely to have caries when compared to African refugees, and they were 4.7 times more likely to have unmet dental needs despite having more access to dentists in their home countries [8]. Ogawa and colleagues noted the same protective factors and low rates of caries for refugees from Africa more than ten years later [6]. These variations among groups highlight the importance of understanding the role of early health experiences and risk factors for dental caries which can be geographically associated.

Other factors can contribute to specific oral health patterns in certain refugee and immigrant groups. Children from East African countries, in particular, have been found to be naturally exposed to optimal or even high levels of fluoride in water supplies [6,8]. Further, East African children from Somalia and Ethiopia are raised on a traditional diet that is very low in sugar and have cultural practices, such as the use of chewing sticks, that tend to spare them from high rates of caries [6–8]. Children from Eastern European countries have the opposite experience with low rates of fluoride found in water sources and high rates of dental disease [8]. There are also variations within countries that may increase caries risk dependent on family socioeconomic status with children from urban areas and more affluent families exhibiting higher rates of caries because of increased access to sweets and sugary beverages [7,8]. Knowledge of regional variations in the incidence of caries and other cultural factors that impact oral health can help to tailor health messaging to be more effective.

3. Role of Acculturation

Arrival in the United States is a time of stress and adjustment for refugee and immigrant families. Acculturation, defined as "lifestyle and behavioral changes of people as they move from one culture and adapt to another culture, usually as a result of immigration," [9] affects oral health. One of the most significant differences for newly arriving groups in regard to attitudes about oral health is a culture shift to an emphasis on healthy primary teeth. Refugee and immigrant families often arrive from home countries that do not emphasize oral health or even value healthy primary teeth [10–13]. A review of studies on acculturation and the impact on oral health found that in general, increasing acculturation results in improved oral health [9]. Using proxy measures of length of residence and English proficiency reveals improved adherence with preventive dental care for Latino and Chinese immigrant families the longer they reside in the US.

An important aspect that may contribute to slower adoption of health messaging is the common belief of fatalism in certain health outcomes, especially dental caries [11–14]. Many cultures see dental caries as a rite of childhood and there may be no expectation of healthy primary teeth. This knowledge gap affects their belief in the value of preventive dental visits and may predispose already vulnerable populations to increased caries in primary and permanent teeth. Higher-risk communities may benefit from oral health messaging that is tailored within their cultural context and, ideally, presented from members of their own community to build trust and acceptance [14].

Living arrangements for many new arrivals can contribute to poor oral health. Many cultures rely on multigenerational housing with extended family such as grandparents, aunts, uncles and even older siblings providing childcare. Family members who care for young children influence daily routines and food choices, especially bottle use and sweet treats [12]. Many cultures also place great emphasis on respect for older members of their community [13]. Cultural clashes can be seen as families struggle with incorporating health norms from the US that may be at odds with the family elder's belief or opinion. Thus, a grandparent who does not believe in the utility of preventive dental care can be a barrier to accessing care.

In many countries, preventive dental care is not a part of routine healthcare, and this may impact attitudes about when to seek care. One study suggests that Chinese immigrants may first look to homeopathic treatments and consider a dental visit only as a last resort [13]. The common belief that dental care is not necessary if a child is not complaining of pain has been noted in Chinese, Filipino, and African immigrant families [10,11,13], as well as Latinos [8]. One study of West African immigrants found the expense of dental care or insurance to conflict with urgent financial responsibilities related to family members in their home country [10]. Responses to a survey with the same group of West Africans revealed that 10% perceived dental care to be unimportant, with 70% reporting that dental decay was not as urgent a disease as others, such as HIV [10]. For some who did access care, caregivers reported they did so to avoid appearing negligent with local social service agencies [10]. These specific cultural beliefs require detailed conversations and information for families to understand the focus on prevention. Additionally, many refugee and immigrant families qualify for public health insurance programs that provide dental care at low or no cost.

However, a recent US federal government policy change known as the public charge rule may significantly impact utilization of public health insurance programs and, therefore, access to dental services. This policy expands the types of government-funded benefits used to determine whether an immigrant is likely to become primarily dependent on public funding [15]. In particular, health insurance, along with food and housing assistance, will be included in the policy expansion. Though the rule change does not apply to refugees or legal immigrant children under age 21, many families may be confused or fearful that the use of these services may negatively impact their permanent residency application [15,16]. While the rule change is currently being contested in multiple states, barring successful legal rulings, the change will become effective 15 October 2019. By some reports, even the threat of the rule change has already resulted in decreased enrollment in public assistance programs [16].

4. Role of Diet

While multiple factors contribute to the pathophysiology of caries formation, one of the principal causes is dietary sugar intake [7]. Amount and frequency of sugar consumption along with host and environmental factors contribute to caries development. Knowledge gaps regarding risks as well as easy access to processed sugary foods and beverages in the United States result in high sugar diets in immigrant and refugee families. Studies show there is a lack of awareness regarding dietary habits—including unrestricted snacking—that contribute to caries [14,17]. In one study, Mexican-American mothers identified candy and sugary beverages as cariogenic but did not always differentiate the role of carbohydrates in crackers, breads, and cookies [18]. Many newcomer families can benefit from specific information about all sources of excess carbohydrates as they may substitute salty crackers or sweetened yogurt drinks, intending to give their child healthier food options.

Prolonged bottle use is common in certain cultures and is extremely prevalent in Latino and Asian families. Beginning in infancy, immigrant and refugee groups may perceive that infant formula is more convenient [11] or more nutritious [12]. These health beliefs may cause families to choose to feed their children formula over breastfeeding and to bottle-feed for longer periods than recommended. One study showed that 36.8% of Mexican-American children were still drinking from a bottle at 24–48 months of age [19]. This rate was more than double the rate of White and African-American children [19]. In fact, in Latino households, it is typical to calm a crying toddler with bottle of sweetened milk or juice [12,18]. As mentioned previously, since many immigrant households tend to be multifamily or multigenerational, it may be a priority to manage a crying child who keeps others awake. Consequently, giving specific messages about the risks of prolonged bottle feeding with sugary liquids including cow's milk and juice, as well as discussing behavior strategies for trained night feeders, is more practical than simply recommending that they stop bottle feeding. Further, it is important to address that shifting to sippy cups if still filled with sugary liquids will not eliminate the risks of caries, as many mothers may assume [18].

5. Role of Culturally Responsive Care

A detailed review of the need for provider diversity as well as patient preference for a culturally-concordant provider is beyond the scope of this article. However, the concept of culturally responsive care has been recognized as integral to effective partnerships with families and can significantly impact care delivery [14]. Culturally responsive care is healthcare that accepts that the patient's home culture is important and affects the way individuals interact with health systems [20]. An additional barrier that may shape dental care access is that immigrant and refugee groups may lack trust in dental providers, and many endorse fear from dental experiences in their home country, which may contribute to lower use of preventive dental services [13]. Working with diverse populations requires insight into cultural beliefs and practices [13], as well as history of health experiences. Acknowledging that providers have their own culture and biases that may affect patient encounters is another important aspect of culturally responsive care.

Though taking into account all of the nuances of culturally responsive care is important, lack of English proficiency remains a significant barrier to healthcare access [21]. Patients with language barriers have difficulty accessing services and are vulnerable to higher rates of adverse health outcomes [21]. Utilizing the 2007 National Survey of Children's health, Avila and Bramlett found that the largest health disparities were seen for Hispanic children who were recent arrivals and those children living in non-English speaking households [22]. This is critically important since, according to 2017 Pew Research, Mexican immigrants in the US have the lowest rates of English proficiency of any ethnic group [3]. Immigrants from Europe, Canada, Sub-Saharan Africa, and the Middle East have the highest rates of English proficiency [3]. Addressing language barriers with trained medical interpreters is a best practice that is legally mandated in hospitals that receive federal funding [21]. Professional language interpretation should be made available in all healthcare settings.

Dental education has incorporated culturally responsive care as a requirement for training [23]. Dental education is shifting to a multidisciplinary approach that emphasizes the humanistic side of patient care as the foundation of understanding. Overlaying the complex interplay of the patient's individual culture combined with societal influence and acculturation provides a more complete appreciation of the patient and their view of oral health. In their paper, Donate-Bartfield and colleagues emphasized the importance of presenting education on behavioral and ethical concepts that value patient autonomy over historical paternalism [23]. These educational concepts are more effective when introduced prior to community-based learning experiences where dental students care for culturally-diverse patients. Service-learning assignments are an excellent way for students to practice compassionate care while still in an educational setting [14].

Medical schools and health systems have also tried to address cultural insensitivity as well as the racial bias and stereotyping that has impacted health equity for many years [24–27]. Efforts have included medical school and residency curriculum on the care of minority populations and the effects of health disparities [25]. The Office of Minority Health has developed standards for healthcare delivery that is culturally and linguistically sensitive [24]. The standards include a variety of initiatives including a requirement that oral and written notices be printed in multiple languages, developing recruitment strategies for diverse professional as well as support staff, regular educational programming for clinic and hospital personnel, as well as procedures to address cross-cultural conflicts [24]. These standards represent a framework to help build an awareness of the influence of culture on behaviors and access to healthcare.

6. Conclusions

Multiple factors influence the development of dental caries and oral health problems in immigrant and refugee children. Knowledge of protective factors as well as the important role culture plays in the way different ethnic communities interact with health systems can help improve outcomes for high risk populations. Healthcare providers in all disciplines should strive to build therapeutic relationships with at-risk populations and deliver care that is culturally appropriate and can address oral health disparities.

To improve the oral health of immigrant and refugee children, medical providers should:

(1) Ask about diet, specifically about exposure to cariogenic foods and drinks, bottle use, and history of dental care;
(2) Examine the teeth of immigrant and refugee children assessing for white spot lesions and frank decay;
(3) Apply fluoride varnish during primary care visits;
(4) Counsel families on the importance of daily oral hygiene practices, use and amount of fluoridated toothpaste, and encourage fluoridated tap water;
(5) Refer with appropriate urgency to dental providers in your community.

Funding: This research received no external funding.

Acknowledgments: The author would like to thank Delta Dental and Diana B. Cutts for editorial assistance.

Conflicts of Interest: The author declares no conflict of interest.

References

1. Colby, S.L.; Ortman, J.M. *Projections of the Size and Composition of the U.S. Population: 2014 to 2060*; Current Population Reports, P25-1143; U.S. Census Bureau: Washington, DC, USA, 2014.
2. Zong, J.; Batalova, J.; Burrows, M. Frequently Requested Statistics on Immigrants and Immigration in the United States. 14 March 2019. Updated 10 July 2019. Available online: https://www.migrationpolicy.org/article/frequently-requested-statistics-immigrants-and-immigration-united-states#Now (accessed on 7 August 2019).
3. Radford, J. Key Findings about U.S. Immigrants. Pew Research Center. 17 June 2019. Available online: https://www.pewresearch.org/fact-tank/2019/06/03/key-findings-about-u-s-immigrants/ (accessed on 4 June 2019).
4. Older People Projected to Outnumber Children for First Time in U.S. History 13 March 2018. Revised 6 September 2018. Available online: https://www.census.gov/newsroom/press-releases/2018/cb18-41-population-projections.html (accessed on 19 June 2019).
5. Fleming, E.; Afful, J. *Prevalence of Total and Untreated Dental Caries among Youth: United States, 2015–2016*; NCHS Data Brief, no 307; National Center for Health Statistics: Hyattsville, MD, USA, 2018.
6. Ogawa, J.T.; Kiang, J.; Watts, D.J.; Hirway, P.; Lewis, C. Oral Health and Dental Clinic Attendance in Pediatric Refugees. *Pediatr. Dent.* **2019**, *41*, 31–34. [PubMed]
7. Holm, A.K. Diet and Caries in High-Risk Groups in Developed and Developing Countries. *Caries Res.* **1990**, *24* (Suppl. 1), 44–52. [CrossRef] [PubMed]
8. Cote, S.; Geltman, P.; Nunn, M.; Lituri, K.; Henshaw, M.; Garcia, R.I. Dental Caries of Refugee Children Compared with US Children. *Pediatrics* **2004**, *114*, e733. [CrossRef] [PubMed]
9. Gao, X.L.; McGrath, C. A Review of the Oral Health Impacts of Acculturation. *J. Immigr. Minor. Health* **2011**, *13*, 202–213. [CrossRef] [PubMed]

10. Obeng, C.S. Culture and dental health among African immigrant school-aged children in the United States. *Health Educ.* **2007**, *107*, 343–350. [CrossRef]
11. Tiwari, T.; Albino, J. Acculturation and Pediatric Minority Oral Health Interventions. *Dent. Clin.* **2017**, *61*, 549–563. [CrossRef] [PubMed]
12. Ng, M.W. Multicultural influences on child-rearing practices: Implications for today's pediatric dentist. *Pediatr. Dent.* **2003**, *25*, 19–22. [PubMed]
13. Hilton, I.V.; Stephen, S.; Barker, J.C.; Weintraub, J.A. Cultural factors and children's oral health care: A qualitative study of carers of young children. *Community Dent. Oral Epidemiol.* **2007**, *35*, 429–438. [CrossRef] [PubMed]
14. Garcia, R.I.; Cadoret, C.A.; Henshaw, M. Multicultural Issues in Oral Health. *Dent. Clin. N. Am.* **2008**, *52*, 319–332. [CrossRef] [PubMed]
15. Immigrant Legal Resource Center. Public Charge. Available online: https://www.ilrc.org/public-charge (accessed on 26 August 2019).
16. Dewey, C. Immigrants are Going Hungry so Trump Won't Deport Them. *The Washington Post*. 16 March 2017. Available online: https://www.washingtonpost.com/news/wonk/wp/2017/03/16/immigrants-are-now-canceling-their-food-stamps-for-fear-that-trump-will-deport-them/?utm_term=.99340832c097 (accessed on 28 August 2019).
17. Chomitz, V.R.; Park, H.J.; Koch-Weser, S.; Chui, K.K.H.; Sun, L.; Malone, M.E.; Palmer, C.; Loo, C.Y.; Must, A. Modifying dietary risk behaviors to prevent obesity and dental caries in very young children: Results of the Baby Steps to Health pediatric dental pilot. *J. Public Health Dent.* **2019**. [CrossRef] [PubMed]
18. Hoeft, K.S.; Barker, J.C.; Masterson, E.E. Urban Mexican-American mothers' belief about caries etiology in children. *Community Dent. Oral Epidemiol.* **2010**, *38*, 244–255. [CrossRef] [PubMed]
19. Brotanek, J.M.; Halterman, J.S.; Auinger, P.; Flores, G.; Weitzman, M. Iron deficiency, prolonged bottle-feeding and racial-ethnic disparities in young children. *Arch. Pediatr. Adolesc. Med.* **2005**, *159*, 1038–1042. [CrossRef] [PubMed]
20. Carteret, M. Cross-Cultural Values of Latino Families. Dimensions of Culture. 2008. Available online: https://www.dimensionsofculture.com/2010/10/576/ (accessed on 6 August 2019).
21. Goenka, P. Lost in translation: Impact of language barriers on children's healthcare. *Curr. Opin. Pediatr.* **2016**, *28*, 659–666. [CrossRef] [PubMed]
22. Avila, R.M.; Bramlett, M.D. Language and Immigrant Status Effects on Disparities in Hispanic Children's Health Status and Access to Health Care. *Matern. Child Health J.* **2013**, *17*, 415–423. [CrossRef] [PubMed]
23. Donate-Bartfield, E.; Lobb, W.K.; Roucka, T.M. Teaching Culturally Sensitive Care to Dental Students: A Multidisciplinary Approach. *J. Dent. Educ.* **2014**, *78*, 454–464. [PubMed]
24. Chin, J.L. Culturally competent health care. *Public Health Rep.* **2000**, *115*, 25–33. [CrossRef] [PubMed]
25. Van Ryn, M.; Burke, J. The effect of patient race and socioeconomic status on physicians' perceptions of patients. *Soc. Sci. Med.* **2000**, *50*, 813–828. [CrossRef]
26. Peña Dolhun, E.; Muñoz, C.; Grumbach, K. Cross-Cultural Education in U.S. Medical Schools: Development of an Assessment Tool. *Acad. Med.* **2003**, *78*, 615–622. [CrossRef] [PubMed]
27. Geiger, H.J.; Borchelt, G. Racial and ethnic disparities in US health care. *Lancet* **2003**, *362*, 1674. [CrossRef]

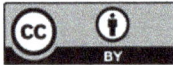

© 2019 by the author. Licensee MDPI, Basel, Switzerland. This article is an open access article distributed under the terms and conditions of the Creative Commons Attribution (CC BY) license (http://creativecommons.org/licenses/by/4.0/).

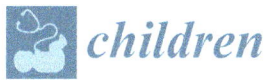

Review

Applying Trauma-Informed Practices to the Care of Refugee and Immigrant Youth: 10 Clinical Pearls

Kathleen K. Miller *, Calla R. Brown, Maura Shramko and Maria Veronica Svetaz

Department of General Pediatrics and Adolescent Health, University of Minnesota, 717 Delaware St SE, Minneapolis, MN 55414, USA
* Correspondence: mill8624@umn.edu; Tel.: +1-319-621-1436

Received: 23 July 2019; Accepted: 14 August 2019; Published: 20 August 2019

Abstract: Immigrant and refugee youth have higher rates of trauma than youth who are not transnational. While youth are incredibly resilient, trauma and toxic stress can result in poor health outcomes that persist throughout life. However, clinical interventions can promote resilience and decrease the negative impact of trauma. This article will review the principles of trauma-informed care and its application for the care of immigrant and refugee youth and their families by sharing concrete and feasible strategies for primary care providers and systems.

Keywords: youth; refugee; immigrant; trauma; health care

1. Introduction

The past decades have seen increasing rates of migration for children and families across international borders. In 2017, as many as 30 million children and youth under the age of 18 were forcibly displaced. Seventeen million of these youth experienced violence or conflict in their home country, and approximately 13 million were eligible for refugee status [1]. Many of these children experienced significant trauma prior to migration, through civil war or unrest, destructive effects of climate change, gang or drug related violence, or poverty [2]. Children are also vulnerable during the migration journey and may be the victims of physical or sexual abuse, unsafe travel conditions, separation from family members, and trafficking [2]. Furthermore, upon arrival in new countries, immigrant youth and families may experience xenophobia and discrimination [3–5]. While these youth possess enormous resilience and strength, the experiences of repeated and prolonged exposure to trauma place them at risk for adverse health outcomes. Trauma and toxic stress are associated with higher rates of depression, anxiety, post-traumatic stress syndrome (PTSD), heart disease, metabolic syndrome, and early death [6–8].

No matter where a clinician is practicing in the world, taking care of children and youth who are immigrants or refugees means caring for children and youth that may have experienced trauma. It is well known that health care centers and primary care providers play a crucial role in promoting resiliency and mitigating the negative outcomes of trauma for immigrant and refugee families [9–11]. The American Academy of Pediatrics recommends utilizing trauma-informed care (TIC) practices when working with immigrant and refugee families [12]. However, it can be challenging to implement these practices without a clear framework and tangible strategies. This article will provide a brief and practical review of TIC and 10 concrete and feasible clinical pearls for promoting a trauma-informed practice with this population.

2. What Is Trauma-Informed Care?

Trauma is defined as "an event, series of events, or set of circumstances that is experienced by an individual as physically or emotionally harmful or life-threatening and that has lasting adverse effects on the individual's functioning and mental, physical, social, emotional, or spiritual well-being" [13]. In the context of pediatric care, TIC is an approach that recognizes the pervasive impact of trauma on children's development and health (as well more broadly throughout systems of service delivery), applies this knowledge of trauma and its consequence into practice, and actively seeks to prevent re-traumatization [13–16]. It is often considered a lens through which to view and interpret child health and outcomes, rather than a specific set of directives. Principles of TIC include promoting physical and psychological safety for patients, building trusting relationships with patients and families, providing peer support, collaborating with patients and families, supporting and fostering agency, and promoting intersectionality [9,12]. Both the American Academy of Pediatrics and the Budapest Declaration on the Rights, Health, and Well-Being of Children and Youth on the Move have identified TIC as a best practice in the care of immigrant and refugee youth [8,13,17].

TIC can be challenging to implement as it is a philosophical approach to care that often encompasses multiple systems and disciplines that were not designed to acknowledge or address experiences of trauma. In this article, we offer 10 clinical pearls to serve as suggestions for starting points to promote TIC for immigrant and refugee families. While not comprehensive, these steps include concrete steps for primary care providers and clinics to support the implementation of TIC.

3. Ten Clinical Pearls for Applying a Trauma-Informed Approach to Care for Refugee and Immigrant Youth

3.1. Practice a Strengths-Based Approach to Care

Although many immigrant and refugee youth have experienced adversity and hardship, first and foremost, they are people who have also drawn on significant internal and external strengths to have survived their past experiences. A critical first step in TIC is to recognize and treat immigrant and refugee children as such. Children are inherently resilient, and immigrant and refugee youth may additionally draw on community and ethnic resiliency [18]. TIC acknowledges and promotes their strengths, resiliency, and capacity to heal from trauma [11,12]. In contrast to a deficit-focused approach, a strengths-based approach focuses on growth and development and recognizes that acknowledging strengths can build resilience and promote healing [19]. The simple act of identifying and drawing attention to children's strengths can promote resilience and additionally serves to identify key family supports. Examples of incorporating a strengths-based approach in a clinical visit are shown in Table 1. Soliciting information about strengths also gives the practitioner insight regarding the youth's sense of self and family dynamics. For example, if a youth struggles to think of anything they are proud of or good at, reinforcing positive parenting practices with parents or caregivers can help build resilience for that child. At times, especially for youth who have experienced trauma without the protective buffering of a caring adult, it may be difficult to identify strengths, and encouraging youth to recognize strengths such as listening skills, sports, reading, helping with childcare or household tasks, or even playing video games, can help re-frame their experiences to validate internal assets. It is important to acknowledge and validate hardships while also exploring and celebrating the youth's role in overcoming adversity.

Table 1. Strengths-based approach to care: clinical examples.

Clinical Skill	Example
Lead the social history or psychosocial assessment with questions about family and patient strengths	"Tell me a little bit about yourself. What are some things that you're really proud of?" "What is something you're good at?"
Gather information about family supports, and strengthen those relationships when possible	"If something difficult were to happen, who would be available to help?" "If something really good were to happen, who would be cheering for you?"
Congratulate patients and families on progress or accomplishments	"I'm so glad to hear that you are smoking fewer cigarettes—that's wonderful! That's a really challenging task. I can tell that you really care about your kids and are motivated to get their asthma under control. You should be really proud of your hard work."
Acknowledge specific strengths, without stereotyping or making assumptions about religious, ethnic, or cultural groups	"That's pretty great that you speak both English and Spanish. It's a huge advantage when looking for jobs or applying to college—make sure to put that on all your applications." "It sounds like your extended family is very close. I'm glad you have so much support available—it's really important when taking care of your children and yourself. You should be proud of all the effort you've put into keeping those relationships strong."
Help patients and families build on past success to continue to build resilience	"It sounds like it was really challenging to cut out soda for the whole family, but you've done it for a whole month now! That is really going to set a healthy example for your kids. What would be another step that you could take as a family to help Dad manage his diabetes?"

3.2. Create an Immigrant-Friendly Healthcare Environment

A critical component of TIC is preventing re-traumatization. Unfortunately, health care environments can be a source of trauma, racism, and xenophobia for immigrants. As a healthcare provider, one way to prevent re-traumatization is by advocating for safe and inclusive environments, including within your own clinic. The process of developing trust starts as soon as a patient interacts with the health care environment. Patients' experiences in the waiting area, check-in desk, and rooming processes all present opportunities to feel welcome or rejected. An inclusive and immigrant-friendly healthcare environment requires regular and ongoing training for all staff that work in a clinic or hospital. The physical environment can also help to promote a sense of welcome. This can be done through the use of signs such as "All Are Welcome Here" posters or signage in multiple languages. Encouraging the hiring of providers and clinic staff who reflect the community being served is another important step in the creation of an inclusive environment [20].

Depending on your location of practice, you may have to consider safety planning in your clinic in the event of an immigration raid. For example, considering what information to document in the medical record about a patient's legal or immigration status or what the clinic staff will do in the case of immigration police presence ahead of time can help to protect your patients [21]. Familiarity with legal requirements when working with immigration enforcement officers, such as articles from the National Immigration Law Center for health care providers in the United States [22], assist providers in knowing what information is protected to avoid unintentionally sharing information that may result in harm to patients or families.

3.3. Promote Trusting Relationships Within the Health Care Environment

One of the fundamental principles of TIC is the importance of trusting relationships and the knowledge that relationships are protective buffers against toxic stress. Primary care providers, in particular, have enormous potential to increase a patient's sense of safety in their health care home. In addition to creating an immigrant friendly clinic, it is important to recognize an individual provider's role in developing trust and rapport. One of the essential components of healing is the creation of safe spaces in which everyone, from parents to children and youth, feels welcome. Empathy and motivational interviewing are critically important tools in establishing this safety. Acknowledge the steps the family or youth have taken in entering into a new and unfamiliar system. The fact that a family has arrived in the exam room is a big step, often in spite of multiple barriers that families have to overcome even before we meet them. Triaging needs according to urgency can continue to develop trust and rapport. It is imperative to allow the patient and family to drive the agenda as much as possible. For example, if a youth is suffering from severe depression or anxiety, counseling about routine health care maintenance may be more effective if done after the patient's mental health has been stabilized and urgent needs met. Of note, the model of trust and mutual respect as an equal partnership between patient and provider is a relatively new development and may be unfamiliar to patients and families. This model of care is a concept worth discussing to allow families and youth to understand that, in this model, they play an important role in making decisions about interventions and health care decisions.

The families of refugee and immigrant youth in your office likely have extensive experience with the health care system in their country of origin, which may be very different from the setting in which you are seeing the patient. The pathways for accessing care, the cost of care, and the methods for receiving results may be barriers for the receipt of health services. Knowing when to utilize an after-hours urgent care or emergency department rather than a primary care office is one example: this may be an unfamiliar model to many families, and education about the role of the primary care office may prevent unnecessary emergency department visits.

Health providers can help to mitigate some of these barriers by intentionally providing education about the healthcare system, including how to access primary care or what to do in case of an emergency, the role of specialists, and how to pick up medications. Seeking help from colleagues such as social workers, patient advocates, or support groups can be extremely useful in helping families navigate the new system [12,23].

3.4. Ask for Permission to Discuss Potentially Difficult Subjects

A trauma-informed approach acknowledges that youth and families can be re-traumatized if they are forced to prematurely share information about traumatic events. Therapists working with victims of trauma often refer to the "window of tolerance": that is, the practice of sharing emotions within a tolerable range [24]. Exceeding the window of tolerance too quickly can result in unacceptable levels of emotional pain and is unlikely to be therapeutic. Borrowing from principles of motivational interviewing, we recommend asking patients and families for permission to discuss sensitive topics [25]. This places the youth in control of their own narrative and allows them to avoid sharing details until they are ready. Ideally, providers should share with the patient why they are asking for information, followed by a request to ask additional questions. For example, "I want to make sure that we're giving you the best medical care possible. In order to make sure I understand your history, I would like to ask a few additional questions about what happened when you were apart from your family. Is that okay with you?"

A similar approach should be utilized with invasive physical examinations. For example, if a pelvic exam is necessary due to clinical concerns, explain the need for the exam and ask for the child or adolescent's permission to perform the exam. Explain that the child can ask the examiner to stop at any time [25]. If a child is unable to tolerate or assent to a physical exam after the procedure has

3.5. Recognize the Impact of Trauma on the Developing Brain, Various Manifestations of Trauma, and Screen for Trauma and Associated Mental Health Conditions

An important aspect of TIC is acknowledgement of the pervasive impact of trauma, including screening for past experiences of trauma. Depression, anxiety, behavioral issues, and PTSD are associated with trauma and have higher prevalence in immigrant and refugee youth than their counterparts who have not experienced similar processes of acculturation or discrimination [26–28]. Immigrant and refugee youth are also less likely than their peers to access health care and preventive services [29], increasing the likelihood of poor outcomes. Unfortunately, literature has shown that immigrant and minority youth are less likely to be screened for depression than their native-born or White counterparts [30]. Ensuring access to quality screening can promote access to effective treatments. Use validated tools for screening for depression and anxiety, such as the Patient Health Questionnare-9 (PHQ-9) [31], Generalized Anxiety Disorder 7-item scale (GAD) [32], or Screen for Child Anxiety-Related Emotional Disorders (SCARED) [33] tools. These tools also have evidence suggesting they are effective for diverse populations and in a variety of languages [34–39]. There are surveys that screen for post-traumatic stress disorder (PTSD), such as the abbreviated UCLA PTSD Reaction Index; however, children rarely meet the full criteria for PTSD, as the criteria has been derived from adult populations [40,41]. Whenever possible, administer surveys in the patient's first language. Finally, screening for sleep problems is essential because of the detrimental effects of trauma on sleep patterns [42].

Additionally, acknowledge the role of previous coping strategies on child and adolescent behavior and development. Youth who have experienced trauma use coping mechanisms to manage chronic stress. These coping mechanisms may have even been adaptive and even necessary for survival in prior circumstances, especially for youth who have experienced extreme violence. However, under less life-threatening circumstances, the coping mechanisms that have served the youth well in the past may create difficulties in the new environment [43,44]. Due to these coping mechanisms, it is wise to consider trauma in the differential diagnosis of youth presenting with behavioral concerns [45,46]. Externalizing behaviors associated with trauma are frequently misdiagnosed as ADHD or ODD. Pharmacological treatment for ADHD or ODD may not be effective or appropriate for the treatment of trauma-related behavioral challenges; thus, it is important to screen for trauma in order to offer proper management and treatment. It can be difficult to differentiate the cognitive impairment associated with chronic stress, anxiety, or depression from ADHD [45]. Therefore, if a diagnosis is in doubt and treatments have been ineffective, referring for an in-depth psychiatric assessment can often provide clarity.

Note that if a family or youth shares stories of trauma, it is important to validate their experiences and emotions and take the necessary time to follow-up positive screens or shared stories.

The list below includes experiences of trauma that may be more prevalent in immigrant and refugee families.

Potential sources of trauma for immigrant and refugee youth

- Anxiety about the possibility of parental deportation or safety of family members in the country or origin;
- Family separation, either planned separation due to immigration logistics or separation as a result of immigration policy or detention;
- Bullying or victimization at school;
- Physical or sexual abuse;
- Dangerous conditions during migration;
- Family conflict or intrafamilial violence;
- Unsafe neighborhoods or gun violence (in country of origin and after relocation);

- Racism and microaggressions (both in country of origin and after relocation).

3.6. Treat Trauma-Related Disorders Appropriately

TIC requires treating trauma. While the evidence-based guidelines for the medical management of trauma and associated disorders are beyond the scope of this article, a brief summary of initial treatment for trauma and its symptoms is provided. Health promotion can be utilized to downregulate the stress response system, for example encouraging habits such as good sleep hygiene, nutritious eating, regular physical activity, play, and engaging with social support systems [41,46]. There is good evidence that trauma-focused cognitive behavioral therapy and child–parent psychotherapy are effective [41]. Medications for depression, anxiety, and sleep difficulty can be utilized as appropriate, and referrals made for care outside of the primary provider's scope of practice. Ideally, the primary care office can serve as a behavioral health home with integrated mental health practitioners and "warm handoffs" to trusted providers [6,23]. When this is not possible, ensure that children are referred to trustworthy providers who have experience in TIC.

Note that diagnoses of depression or anxiety may be stigmatizing to patients, particularly in certain immigrant communities. Framing depression or anxiety as a result of trauma can sometimes help families better understand these disorders; for example, utilize the phrase "stress- and trauma-related disorder" to explain the root symptoms being treated. Qualifiers such as anxiety or depression can used as secondary diagnoses, with an explanation for youth and parents regarding how these symptoms are the result of "what happened to you" rather than "what's wrong with you."

In the treatment of trauma and related mental health disorders, foster agency in youth by asking about their treatment preferences. Whenever possible, give them options in choosing their care. If their preferred treatment option is safe, allow it to the extent possible. Ensure that patients know how to contact the clinic or seek follow-up or emergency care.

3.7. Utilize a Two-Generational Approach to Care

When children and youth completed the transnational journey with most of the close family, remember that each individual of the family has experienced the same traumatic events (war, extreme poverty, persecution, etc.). Parents and caretakers can offer one of the most protective factors for children and adolescents in surviving stress and trauma and supportive and consistent relationships with a caring adult can buffer youth from the negative impacts of trauma [14,26,46]. Given the role parents and caretakers play in the management of childhood trauma, healthcare providers should extend their triage to caregivers. Support caregivers in navigating a new and unfamiliar health care system in order to ensure that they are able to access the same care the youth is receiving by working with ancillary services, such as social workers or community mental health practitioners.

Youth and children often lose the adult protection that caregivers provided in their country of origin. Children and youth experience "adultification" as they learn the new rules of a culture and master language skills more quickly than their caregivers [47,48]. Children then run the risk of becoming the internal cultural brokers of the family. Providers need to be aware of these dynamics and recognize the anxiety it can cause in youth. Depression may also result from feelings of loss of parental efficacy that parents and caregivers may experience. For example, parents and caregivers may have been stripped of the privileges afforded to them in their country of origin (such as fluency in the primary language, professional status, or primary breadwinner). These losses can have significant effects on parental or caregiver mental health and, by extension, on the health of children and adolescents.

Immigrant and refugee parents often need more coaching during their child's adolescence than would have been necessary if they were living in their country of origin. As these parents did not complete the majority of their developmental growth in the host country, they can feel lost or disoriented when guiding their adolescence through their teenage years in an unfamiliar environment. Additionally, the new culture may foster more individualistic behaviors than the country of origin, which can result in a clash of values between an adolescent seeking independence and parents seeking to protect their children and promote community-oriented values [48].

3.8. Know Your Own Local Resources and Make Sure They Are Trustworthy

Partnerships with other individuals and agencies in your area outside of health care can be an invaluable resource for TIC with refugee and immigrant youth. Immigrant and refugee youth and their families may have past experiences of trauma that impact their trust or engagement with various services and may be unfamiliar with how to access services in an unfamiliar environment. Healthcare providers may be the first professionals to interact with immigrants and refugee youth and families and as such can play a vital role in bridging interrelated systems and services. These can include experts in your own country's immigration law, counselors and psychologists practicing trauma-informed mental health care in the youth or caregivers' first language, community centers for community building and physical activity, and resources for nutritious food and safe housing. Legal assistance in particular can be helpful if immigrants are undocumented [9,12]. Children and adolescents who live with undocumented family members have been shown to have high anxiety levels about the fear of deportation of family members [49,50], and lack of documentation can result in additional barriers to care that result in poorer health outcomes [51–53]. Thus, it is important to refer to low-cost or free legal services to promote health for the entire family.

3.9. Recognize that Trauma May Not End after Migration

In an ideal world, all youth on the move would not be exposed to new trauma once the migration journey is complete. However, it is important to acknowledge that trauma in the form of racism, bias, and microaggressions may continue long after migration [4,28,54]. Chronic exposure to racism has been associated with negative long-term health outcomes [20,55] and with perceived poor quality of medical care [4]. This relationship can be explored with your patients using the principles of TIC. As most youth will spend a majority of their time in educational environments, it is important to screen for bullying, racism, and victimization at school. Finally, this can be an opportunity to explore the youth's resilience mechanisms, emphasizing the unique cultural strengths of the individual and family, including conversations about racism and cultural socialization.

3.10. Advocate for Your Patients Both in and outside the Clinic: For Your Patients and for Yourself

Using principles of TIC can provide safety for families and promote recovery, but it is also important to recognize that the act of caring for traumatized youth can be difficult and may lead to secondary traumatic stress. For health care providers on the front line of listening to patients' stories, community advocacy is a strategy to transform secondary trauma, grief, and anger into action. Healthcare providers are well respected members of society in many communities and as such have unique privileges and power and are also uniquely positioned to listen to their patients' stories directly. Using this power and knowledge to push for immigrant-friendly policies, a diverse healthcare workforce, and anti-racist policies can allow for health care providers to harness emotions to action. Healthcare providers are in an ideal position to write editorials for local and national news outlets, write letters to governing representatives, testify before local and national legislators, and organize within professional governing bodies to advocate for best practices for the care of immigrant and refugee families.

4. Conclusions

This discussion of TIC for refugee and immigrant youth is far from exhaustive. However, these clinical pearls can provide a concrete framework for incorporating a trauma-informed lens to your practice, including in relationship-building, diagnosis, management, and promotion of resilience. Utilizing the principles of TIC can also allow for providers to both recognize and treat experiences of trauma while also seeing beyond the trauma and develop an appreciation for the unique strengths of each patient and family. In turn, applying TIC can help promote well-being and health not just for immigrant and refugee youth and families, but also within our health care system by challenging and improving health care delivery from a trauma-informed perspective more broadly.

Ten Clinical Pearls of Trauma Informed Care for Refugee and Immigrant Youth

1. Practice a strengths-based approach to care;
2. Create an immigrant-friendly healthcare environment;
3. Promote trusting relationships within the healthcare environment;
4. Ask for permission to discuss potentially difficult subjects;
5. Recognize the impact of trauma on the developing brain and various manifestations of trauma and screen for trauma and associated mental health conditions;
6. Treat trauma and its associated symptoms appropriately;
7. Utilize a two-generational approach to care;
8. Know your own local resources and make sure they are trustworthy;
9. Recognize that trauma may not end after migration;
10. Advocate for your patients both in and outside the clinic: for your patients and for yourself.

Author Contributions: Conceptualization, K.K.M., M.S. and C.R.B.; Writing-original draft preparation, K.K.M. and C.R.B.; writing-review and editing, M.V.S. and M.S.; supervision, M.V.S.

Funding: This project was supported by the Health Resources and Services Administration (HRSA) of the US Department of Health and Human Services (HHS) under National Research Service Award in Primary Medical Care grant number T32HP22239 (PI: Borowsky), Bureau of Health Workforce. This information or content and conclusions are those of the author and should not be construed as the official position or policy of, nor should any endorsements be inferred by HRSA, HHS, or the US Government. This work was also conducted as part of the University of Minnesota Leadership Education in Adolescent Health (LEAH) Interdisciplinary Fellowship at the University of Minnesota, funded through the Maternal Child Health Bureau. This project was also supported by the Eliminating Health Disparities Initiative from the Minnesota Department of Health, and Dr. Svetaz would like to thank the initiative for their ongoing support and collaboration.

Acknowledgments: We would like to acknowledge the hundreds to thousands of patients who have entrusted us with their health and shared their journeys, challenges, and triumphs with us. We thank them for the privilege.

Conflicts of Interest: The authors declare no conflict of interest.

References

1. United Nations High Commissioner for Refugees. Global Trends: Forced Displacement in 2017. Available online: https://www.unhcr.org/globaltrends2017/ (accessed on 13 August 2019).
2. UN Department of Economic and Social Affairs. Youth Issue Briefs: Youth and Migration. 2016. Available online: https://www.un.org/esa/socdev/documents/youth/fact-sheets/youth-migration.pdf (accessed on 14 August 2019).
3. Sidhu, S.S. Impact of recent executive actions on minority youth and families. *J. Am. Acad. Child Adolesc. Psychiatry* **2017**, *56*, 805–807. [CrossRef] [PubMed]
4. Perez, D.; Sribney, W.M.; Rodríguez, M.A. Perceived Discrimination and Self-Reported Quality of Care among Latinos in the United States. *J. Gen. Intern. Med.* **2009**, *24*, 548–554. [CrossRef] [PubMed]
5. Oxman-Martinez, J.; Rummens, A.J.; Moreau, J.; Choi, Y.R.; Beiser, M.; Ogilvie, L.; Armstrong, R. Perceived ethnic discrimination and social exclusion: Newcomer immigrant children in Canada. *Am. J. Orthopsychiatry* **2012**, *82*, 376–388. [CrossRef] [PubMed]
6. American Academy of Pediatrics. Adverse Childhood Experiences and the Lifelong Consequences of Trauma. 2014. Available online: https://www.aap.org/en-us/documents/ttb_aces_consequences.pdf (accessed on 12 August 2019).
7. Brown, D.W.; Anda, R.F.; Tiemeier, H.; Felitti, V.J.; Edwards, V.J.; Croft, J.B.; Giles, W.H. Adverse Childhood Experiences and the Risk of Premature Mortality. *Am. J. Prev. Med.* **2009**, *37*, 389–396. [CrossRef] [PubMed]

8. Felitti, V.J.; Anda, R.F.; Nordenberg, D.; Williamson, D.F.; Spitz, A.M.; Edwards, V.; Koss, M.P.; Marks, J.S. Relationship of childhood abuse and household dysfunction to many of the leading causes of death in adults. The Adverse Childhood Experiences (ACE) Study. *Am. J. Prev. Med.* **1998**, *14*, 245–258. [CrossRef]
9. Robinson, L.K. Arrived: The crisis of unaccompanied children at our southern border. *Pediatrics* **2015**, *135*, 205–207. [CrossRef] [PubMed]
10. Huerta, A. Health Care Centers Can Become Safe Spaces for Immigrant Patients. 2017. Available online: https://www.nilc.org/news/the-torch/5-25-17/ (accessed on 12 August 2019).
11. Dawson-Hahn, E.; Cházaro, A. Mitigating the health consequences for youth in families affected by immigration policy changes opportunities for health care professionals and health systems. *JAMA Pediatrics* **2019**. [CrossRef]
12. Linton, J.M.; Griffin, M.; Shapiro, A.J. Detention of immigrant children. *Pediatrics* **2017**, *139*, e20170483. [CrossRef] [PubMed]
13. SAMHSA's Trauma and Justice Strategic Initiative. SAMHSA's Concept of Trauma and Guidance for a Trauma-Informed Approach. 2014. Available online: https://www.nasmhpd.org/sites/default/files/SAMHSA_Concept_of_Trauma_and_Guidance.pdf (accessed on 12 August 2019).
14. Marsac, M.L.; Kassam-Adams, N.; Hildenbrand, A.K.; Nicholls, E.; Winston, F.K.; Leff, S.S.; Fein, J. Implementing a trauma-informed approach in pediatric health care networks. *JAMA Pediatrics* **2016**, *170*, 70–77. [CrossRef] [PubMed]
15. Loomis, B.; Epstein, K.; Dauria, E.F.; Dolce, L. Implementing a trauma-informed public health system in San Francisco, California. *Health Educ. Behav.* **2019**, *46*, 251–259. [CrossRef] [PubMed]
16. American Academy of Pediatrics. *The Medical Home Approach to Identifying and Responding to Exposure to Trauma*; American Academy of Pediatrics: Washington, DC, USA, 2014.
17. International Society for Social Pediatrics and Child Health (ISSOP). Budapest Declaration on the Rights, Health and Well-being of Children and Youth on the Move. October 2017. Available online: https://www.issop.org/cmdownloads/budapest-declaration-on-the-rights-health-and-well-being-of-children-and-youth-on-the-move/ (accessed on 12 August 2019).
18. Neblett, E.W.; Rivas-Drake, D.; Umaña-Taylor, A.J.; Rivas-Drake, D.; Umaña-Taylor, A.J. The Promise of Racial and Ethnic Protective Factors in Promoting Ethnic Minority Youth Development. *Child Dev. Perspect.* **2012**, *6*, 295–303. [CrossRef]
19. Smith, E.J. The Strength-Based Counseling Model. *Couns. Psychol.* **2006**, *34*, 134–144. [CrossRef]
20. The Society for Adolescent Health and Medicine. Racism and its harmful effects on nondominant racial–ethnic youth and youth-serving providers: A call to action for organizational change. *J. Adolesc. Health* **2018**, *63*, 257–261. [CrossRef] [PubMed]
21. Kim, G.; Molina, U.S.; Saadi, A. Should immigration status information be included in a patient's health record? *AMA J. Ethics* **2019**, *21*, 8–16.
22. National Immigration Law Center. Health Care Providers and Immigration Enforcement: Know Your Rights, Know Your Patients' Rights. 2017. Available online: https://www.nilc.org/issues/immigration-enforcement/healthcare-provider-and-patients-rights-imm-enf/ (accessed on 13 July 2019).
23. Clark, C.; Classen, C.C.; Fourt, A.; Maithili, S. *Treating the Trauma Survivor: An Essential Guide to Trauma-Informed Care*, 1st ed.; Routledge: New York, NY, USA, 2015.
24. Reproductive Health Access Project. Contraceptive Pearl: Trauma-Informed Pelvic Exams. 2015. Available online: https://www.reproductiveaccess.org/resource/trauma-informed-pelvic-exams/ (accessed on 13 July 2019).
25. Rollnick, S.; Butler, C.C.; Miller, W.R. *Motivational Interviewing in Health Care*, 1st ed.; The Guilford Press: New York, NY, USA, 2008.
26. Potochnick, S.R.; Perreira, K.M. Depression and Anxiety among First-Generation Immigrant Latino Youth. *J. Nerv. Ment. Dis.* **2010**, *198*, 470–477. [CrossRef] [PubMed]
27. Gee, G.C.; Ryan, A.; Laflamme, D.J.; Holt, J. Self-Reported Discrimination and Mental Health Status Among African Descendants, Mexican Americans, and Other Latinos in the New Hampshire REACH 2010 Initiative: The Added Dimension of Immigration. *Am. J. Public Health* **2006**, *96*, 1821–1828. [CrossRef]
28. Huang, K.Y.; Calzada, E.; Cheng, S.; Brotman, L.M. Physical and mental health disparities among young children of Asian immigrants. *J. Pediatrics* **2012**, *160*, 331.e1–336.e1. [CrossRef]

29. Huang, Z.J.; Yu, S.M.; Ledzra, R. Health Status and Health Service Access and Use among Children in U.S. Immigrant Families. *Am. J. Public Health* **2006**, *96*, 634–640. [CrossRef]
30. Zenlea, I.S.; Milliren, C.E.; Mednick, L.; Rhodes, E.T. Depression screening in adolescents in the United States: A national study of ambulatory, office-based practice. *Acad. Pediatr.* **2014**, *14*, 186–191. [CrossRef]
31. Kroenke, K.; Spitzer, R.L.; Williams, J.B.W. The Patient Health Questionnaire-9: Validity of a brief depression severity measure. *J. Gen. Intern. Med.* **2001**, *16*, 606–613. [CrossRef]
32. Löwe, B.; Decker, O.; Müller, S.; Brähler, E.; Schellberg, D.; Herzog, W.; Herzberg, P.Y. Validation and Standardization of the Generalized Anxiety Disorder Screener (GAD-7) in the General Population. *Med. Care* **2009**, *46*, 266–274. [CrossRef]
33. Birmaher, B.; Khetarpal, S.; Brent, D.; Cully, M.; Balach, L.; Kaufman, J.; Neer, S.M. The Screen for Child Anxiety Related Emotional Disorders (SCARED): Scale construction and psychometric characteristics. *J. Am. Acad. Child Adolesc. Psychiatry* **1997**, *36*, 545–553. [CrossRef]
34. Mills, S.D.; Fox, R.S.; Malcarne, V.L.; Roesch, S.C.; Champagne, B.R.; Sadler, G.R. The psychometric properties of the Generalized Anxiety Disorder-7 scale in Hispanic Americans with English or Spanish language preference. *Cult. Divers. Ethn. Minor. Psychol.* **2014**, *20*, 463–468. [CrossRef]
35. Garcia-Campayo, J.; Zamorano, E.; Ruiz, M.; Pardo, A.; Freire, Ó.; Pérez-Páramo, M.; López-Gómez, V.; Rejas, J. P01-150 Cultural adaptation into Spanish of the generalized anxiety disorder scale-7 (GAD-7) scale. *Eur. Psychiatry* **2009**, *24*, S538. [CrossRef]
36. Wang, W.; Bian, Q.; Zhao, Y.; Li, X.; Wang, W.; Du, J.; Zhang, G.; Zhou, Q.; Zhao, M. Reliability and validity of the Chinese version of the Patient Health Questionnaire (PHQ-9) in the general population. *Gen. Hosp. Psychiatry* **2014**, *36*, 539–544. [CrossRef] [PubMed]
37. Monahan, P.O.; Shacham, E.; Reece, M.; Kroenke, K.; Ong'or, W.O.; Omollo, O.; Yebei, V.N.; Ojwang, C. Validity/reliability of PHQ-9 and PHQ-2 depression scales among adults living with HIV/AIDS in Western Kenya. *J. Gen. Intern. Med.* **2009**, *24*, 189–197. [CrossRef] [PubMed]
38. Essau, C.A.; Anastassiou-Hadjicharalambous, X.; Muñoz, L.C. Psychometric properties of the screen for child anxiety related emotional disorders (SCARED) in Cypriot children and adolescents. *Eur. J. Psychol. Assess.* **2013**, *29*, 19–28. [CrossRef]
39. Su, L.; Wang, K.; Fan, F.; Su, Y.; Gao, X. Reliability and validity of the screen for child anxiety related emotional disorders (SCARED) in Chinese children. *J. Anxiety Disord.* **2008**, *22*, 612–621. [CrossRef]
40. Cohen, J.A.; Kelleher, K.J.; Mannarino, A.P. Identifying, treating, and referring traumatized children. *Arch. Pediatr. Adolesc. Med.* **2008**, *162*, 447. [CrossRef]
41. Copeland, W.E.; Keeler, G.; Angold, A.; Costello, E.J. Traumatic events and posttraumatic stress in childhood. *Arch. Gen. Psychiatry* **2007**, *64*, 577. [CrossRef]
42. Sadeh, A. Stress, trauma, and sleep in children. *Child Adolesc. Psychiatr. Clin. N. Am.* **1996**, *5*, 685–700. [CrossRef]
43. Hunt, T.K.A.; Slack, K.S.; Berger, L.M. Adverse childhood experiences and behavioral problems in middle childhood. *Child Abus. Negl.* **2017**, *67*, 391–402. [CrossRef] [PubMed]
44. Kendall, P.C.; Compton, S.N.; Walkup, J.T.; Birmaher, B.; Albano, A.M.; Sherrill, J.; Ginsburg, G.; Rynn, M.; McCracken, J.; Gosch, E.; et al. Clinical characteristics of anxiety disordered youth. *J. Anxiety Disord.* **2010**, *24*, 360–365. [CrossRef] [PubMed]
45. MacLean, S.A.; Agyeman, P.O.; Walther, J.; Singer, E.K.; Baranowski, K.A.; Katz, C.L. Mental health of children held at a United States immigration detention center. *Soc. Sci. Med.* **2019**, *230*, 303–308. [CrossRef] [PubMed]
46. American Academy of Pediatrics. Trauma Toolbox for Primary Care. 2014. Available online: https://www.aap.org/en-us/advocacy-and-policy/aap-health-initiatives/healthy-foster-care-america/Pages/Trauma-Guide.aspx#trauma (accessed on 12 August 2019).
47. Puig, M.E. The adultification of refugee children. *J. Hum. Behav. Soc. Environ.* **2002**, *5*, 85–95. [CrossRef]
48. Kam, J.A. The Effects of language brokering frequency and feelings on Mexican-heritage youth's mental health and risky behaviors. *J. Commun.* **2011**, *61*, 455–475. [CrossRef]
49. Brabeck, K.; Xu, Q. The Impact of Detention and Deportation on Latino Immigrant Children and Families: A Quantitative Exploration. *Hisp. J. Behav. Sci.* **2010**, *32*, 341–361. [CrossRef]
50. Zayas, L.H.; Aguilar-Gaxiola, S.; Yoon, H.; Rey, G.N. The distress of citizen-children with detained and deported parents. *J. Child Fam. Stud.* **2015**, *24*, 3213–3223. [CrossRef] [PubMed]

51. Vargas, E.D.; Ybarra, V.D. US Citizen children of undocumented parents: The link between state immigration policy and the health of Latino children. *J. Immigr. Minor Heal.* **2017**, *19*, 913–920. [CrossRef] [PubMed]
52. Suárez-Orozco, C. Conferring disadvantage: Behavioral and developmental implications for children growing up in the shadow of undocumented immigration status. *J. Dev. Behav. Pediatr.* **2017**, *38*, 424–428. [CrossRef] [PubMed]
53. Wood, L.C.N. Impact of punitive immigration policies, parent-child separation and child detention on the mental health and development of children. *BMJ Paediatr. Open* **2018**, *2*, e000338. [CrossRef] [PubMed]
54. Lauderdale, D.S.; Wen, M.; Jacobs, E.A.; Kandula, N.R. Immigrant perceptions of discrimination in health care: The California health interview survey 2003. *Med. Care* **2006**, *44*, 914–920. [CrossRef] [PubMed]
55. Williams, D.; Mohamed, S. Discrimination and racial disparities in health: Evidence and needed research. *J. Behav. Med.* **2009**, *32*, 20–47. [CrossRef] [PubMed]

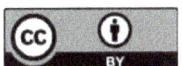

© 2019 by the authors. Licensee MDPI, Basel, Switzerland. This article is an open access article distributed under the terms and conditions of the Creative Commons Attribution (CC BY) license (http://creativecommons.org/licenses/by/4.0/).

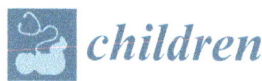

Viewpoint

Refugee and Asylum-Seeking Children: Interrupted Child Development and Unfulfilled Child Rights

Ziba Vaghri [1,*], Zoë Tessier [1] and Christian Whalen [2]

1. School of Public Health and Social Policy, Faculty of Human and Social Development, University of Victoria, Victoria, BC V8P 5C2, Canada; ztessier@uvic.ca
2. Office of Child and Youth Advocate, Fredericton, NB E3B 5H1, Canada; Christian.Whalen@gnb.ca
* Correspondence: zibav@uvic.ca; Tel.: +1-250-472-4900

Received: 22 August 2019; Accepted: 24 October 2019; Published: 30 October 2019

Abstract: The 21st century phenomenon of "global displacement" is particularly concerning when it comes to children. Childhood is a critical period of accelerated growth and development. These processes can be negatively affected by the many stressors to which refugee and asylum-seeking children are subjected. The *United Nations Convention on the Rights of the Child* (*CRC*) is the most ratified human rights treaty in history, with 196 States Parties (SPs). The *CRC* provides a framework of 54 articles outlining government responsibilities to ensure the protection, promotion, and fulfillment of rights of all children within their jurisdictions. Among these are the rights of refugee and asylum-seeking children, declared under Article 22 of the *CRC*. Refugee and asylum-seeking children, similarly to all other children, are entitled to their rights under the *CRC* and do not forgo any right by virtue of moving between borders. The hosting governments, as SPs to the *CRC*, are the primary duty bearers to fulfill these rights for the children entering their country. This manuscript provides an overview of the health and developmental ramification of being displaced for refugee and asylum-seeking children. Then, an in-depth analysis of the provisions under Article 22 is presented and the responsibilities of SPs under this article are described. The paper provides some international examples of strengths and shortcomings relating to these responsibilities and closes with a few concluding remarks and recommendations.

Keywords: Convention on the Rights of the Child; child rights; refugee; asylum-seeking children; child health; child development; Article 22 of the CRC; children on the move

1. Background and Context

The *United Nations Convention on the Rights of the Child* (*CRC*) is the first human rights treaty that has considered a series of unique human rights specifically for children. The *CRC* has recognized this important phase of life as being a period of accelerated growth and development as well as a time of great vulnerability. Therefore, it has made provisions to promote such development (through, for example, provision and participation rights, such as the right to education and freedom of expression) and to prevent harms to which children may be vulnerable (through protection rights) [1]. The *CRC* is the most highly ratified human rights treaty in history, with ratification from all member States of the United Nations (UN), except the United States of America (United States) [2]. Through ratification, countries become States Parties (SPs) to the *CRC* and have the obligation to (a) harmonize their domestic laws and policies with the *CRC* so that internal systems do not contradict any provision, (b) implement all rights articulated under the *CRC* for children within their jurisdiction, and (c) monitor and report the process of implementation of the *CRC* to a Geneva-based committee known as the United Nations Committee on the Rights of the Child (the Committee hereafter) [1].

This year, the global community is celebrating the 30th anniversary of the *CRC*. Three decades have passed since its adoption by the General Assembly in 1989, and yet, the global community continues to face huge challenges in moving past lip service for children and truly protect their many rights as articulated under the *CRC*. While the unprecedented ratification of this treaty, by all UN Member States but one, speaks strongly about the world's unanimity for children's rights, the global community, more often than not, falls short in fulfilling the provisions under the *CRC*. Violations of children's rights have grave ramifications, particularly when they happen in a systemic manner and on a massive scale. Such is the case in relation to the rights of refugee and asylum-seeking children.

Under Article 22 of the *CRC*, a child or young person who leaves their country of origin to escape war, persecution, or natural disaster, has the right to appropriate protection and provisions, such as health, education, and housing. The rights under the *CRC* govern all children regardless of where in the world they are located; thus, refugee and asylum-seeking children do not lose any of their rights simply because they have moved from one country to another [1]. However, in reality, this is not the case and many of these children, depending on where in the world they move to, are denied many of their rights. Often, the host States, who have a clear set of obligations under the *CRC*, fail to fulfill their responsibilities for refugee and asylum-seeking children and by doing so, subject children to a discriminatory treatment. Such discrimination can not only adversely impact children's health and development, but also violate their human rights under the *CRC*.

In this manuscript, we will provide an overview of the ramifications of being displaced for children's health and development and present a critical examination of the rights and provisions under this article. We then outline some international examples of variations in compliance with Article 22 among the host countries, highlighting SPs' strengths and shortcomings. The manuscript closes with concluding remarks and recommendations for improving the monitoring, reporting, and accountability mechanisms to support refugee and asylum-seeking children. Throughout this manuscript, the term "these children" will refer to children who are " ... seeking refugee status or who [are] considered [refugees] in accordance with applicable international or domestic law and procedures, whether unaccompanied or accompanied by [their] parents" under Article 22 of the *CRC*, unless a special sub-category of these children, such as unaccompanied children, are the topic of discussion, in which case they will be identified accordingly [1].

2. Refugee and Asylum-Seeking Children

2.1. The Scope of the Phenomenon

Globally, millions of individuals are currently displaced and seek refuge for various reasons, such as environmental disasters, economic devastation, violation of human rights, and fear of persecution [3]. In 2018, an estimated 13.6 million individuals were newly displaced. This population consisted of 10.8 million people internally displaced, and 2.8 million refugees and asylum-seekers [4]. Worldwide, the total number of individuals that are forcibly displaced reached 70.8 million in 2018. The majority of refugees globally (67%) originated from only five countries: the Syrian Arab Republic, Afghanistan, South Sudan, Myanmar, and Somalia [4]. However, Venezuelan refugee and asylum-seeker movement within and between borders is increasingly problematic, with an estimated 3.4 million individuals displaced outside the country's border in 2018, and numbers projected to increase to an estimated 5 million people by the end of 2019. The five countries that host the most refugees are Pakistan, Uganda, Sudan, Germany, and Turkey [4].

Despite the fact that humanitarian assistance mechanisms are in place, the demand far surpasses the supply. Only a small percentage of refugees are resettled each year, and humanitarian visas are difficult to obtain. In 2017, more than 1.19 million people were in need of resettlement; however, only 170,000 were accommodated [5]. Protection of children when they are displaced and on the move is seriously compromised, as there are few legal, safe migration channels accessible. This pressures children and their families to utilize dangerous and risky means for migration, such as paying migrant smuggling services to circumvent restriction and heavily guarded boarders. An estimated 90% of irregular migrants entering Europe in 2015 used such services at some point during their journey [5].

Although less than 3% of the refugee population returned to their countries of origin in 2018, many of them returned to unsafe conditions unsustainable for the protection of child rights [4].

Approximately half of the overall refugee population are children under the age of 18 years [4]. Unaccompanied and separated children are among the most vulnerable of refugees. These children migrate alone or are accompanied by someone other than a parent or legal guardian. Approximately 111,000 unaccompanied children were reported in 2018, although only 27,600 applied for asylum [4]. Due to challenges in reaching and assessing this population, these figures are likely to be an underestimate. The rights declared under the CRC for refugee and asylum-seeking children are often violated, resulting in significantly adverse impacts on children's health and development, which is already in a fragile and compromised state.

2.2. Health and Development of Displaced Children

Childhood is a period of rapid growth and development in all physical, mental, spiritual, and social domains [6,7]. Despite their importance, protection and promotion of rights during this stage are seriously compromised when it comes to refugee and asylum-seeking children. Prolonged exposure to unfavourable conditions—for example, hunger, limited access to education and health services, low socioeconomic status, and exposure to violence, war, abuse, and exploitation—has lasting effects on a child's ability to thrive [6]. These experiences can be considered as Adverse Childhood Experiences (ACEs). The accumulation of ACEs results in increased negative health outcomes and can have lasting impacts later in life. For example, ACEs are associated with mental health problems (e.g., depression, anxiety, and Post-Traumatic Stress Disorder (PTSD)), chronic conditions (e.g., heart disease, diabetes, cancer), high risk-taking behaviours (e.g., substance abuse and unsafe sexual practices), and lower academic achievement and income well into adulthood [8–10]. Subsequent lifelong adverse health outcomes in different domains of development, are experienced by children undergoing these circumstances before, during, and after seeking asylum [6].

2.2.1. Physical and Mental Health

The physical health of refugee and asylum-seeking children is negatively affected by living conditions, malnutrition, lack of clean water sources, and limited access to medical services [6]. For instance, there is an increased prevalence of infectious diseases, such as tuberculosis, hepatitis B, HIV, and malaria, as well as higher rates of dental caries and poor oral health, resulting from a lack of health and dental services [6,11,12]. Youth reproductive and sexual health is often overlooked, and access to such education is limited [13]. Refugee children are also more likely to suffer from vaccine-preventable diseases due to the sub-optimal immunization coverage in their country of origin or missing follow-up doses of vaccination while they are on the move [14].

Limited resources in refugee camps can result in maladaptive behaviours such as drug and substance abuse. Such behaviours from adults and children can further exacerbate experiences of sexual abuse and exploitation of children in the form of prostitution, child labour, and domestic servitude [15]. These threats to the protection of children have serious consequences for physical and mental health, and lead to other problematic repercussions, such as unwanted pregnancies, sexually transmitted infections, prolonged and/or more serious maladaptive coping behaviours, increased levels of stress, and physical harm, including the child or young person's involvement with gangs or criminal activity [16,17].

Trauma is the common experience of all refugee and asylum-seeking children. Many witness the death of a family member or friend or acts of violence to self and others, and experience traumatic events when fleeing their country of origin. Children can also be victims of sexual violence, various types of abuse, neglect, human trafficking, and military recruitment [18]. Damaging personal experiences can traumatize a child and deeply affect their mental health, which can have direct (as is the case with personal injury or death of family members) and indirect (arising from prolonged lack of education, material deprivation) negative impacts on children's well-being and development [18,19].

Stress and trauma experienced during the risky journey to asylum can later manifest into various long-lasting physical and psychological effects. The presentation of trauma in children can sometimes be difficult to detect but often includes symptoms such as anxiety, mood disorders, depression, sleep disturbances, PTSD, and interpersonal difficulties [20].

Children on the move can also undergo inhumane and harmful detention and can experience lasting emotional and behavioural distress during and after detainment, even if they are housed for a brief period of time [21,22]. Acute as well as chronic stress elevate harmful hormone levels in the body, contribute to chronic health conditions, and are toxic to the developing brain [23]. Many children do not feel safe reporting these predicaments due to a lack of social support and fear that their safety and protection may be further compromised [15].

The trauma of displacement can be compounded by separation from parents or any loss of stable caregivers. Children may be unaccompanied for a number of reasons, such as being sent to claim asylum while the parent stayed behind, separation during the journey, or death of a parent. Neurologically, separation from parents at this critical time can disrupt brain development and impact future physical, emotional, social, and cognitive maturation. Separation, when young, makes children more susceptible to a variety of psychological problems and hinders their ability to make social connections later in life [24]. This prolonged exposure to stress is toxic and can have serious health ramification. Sometimes, the detrimental consequences of such toxic stress can be delayed to later life and manifest themselves in the form of susceptibility to anxiety, mental disorder or predispositions to cancer or other non-communicable diseases [25].

Even when not separated, parents themselves experience trauma and its corresponding consequences as a result of being displaced and on the move. Parents' suffering from a psychological disorder can also influence the child's mental, emotional, and behavioural well-being, a phenomenon called transgenerational transmission of trauma [26]. Both the parents' and child's exposure to trauma disrupts the dynamic of the child-caregiver dyad, negatively affecting attachment and generating expectations of harm, distrust, and poor emotional and social connectivity [20].

Lastly, the predicament of the young fetus in the womb of the refugee and asylum-seeking mother subjected to all the above-mentioned stressors is of grave significance to child development. While history has documented the horrendous assault to humanity during the Holocaust and the Dutch Famine, retrospective studies of individuals who lived through these events during their intra-uterine lives have illustrated extended consequences of these assaults. The surviving fetuses of such experiences have shown to have higher propensity to develop high blood pressure, diabetes, and obesity and genetic tagging for trauma-related disorders [27–29]. A life course approach to child development necessitates awareness of the consequences of traumatic events (e.g., from prolonged periods of displacement and being on the move) and the effects for the developing fetuses of expecting mothers.

2.2.2. Other Social Determinants of Health

Inadequate nutrition and material deprivation are constant components of the predicament of these children. It is important to consider the relationship between socioeconomic status and pre- and post-migration factors. Financial resources affect how efficiently individuals can escape their country of origin, and the food, shelter, and transportation that is accessible during the journey to asylum. Upon arrival, the high-income countries often have the necessary resources to provide refugee children with basic material needs, although other existing challenges affect development and the ability to thrive [22]. For example, unemployment rates are disproportionately higher for refugees than economic migrants or the general population, even years after resettlement. Refugees are also more likely to have temporary jobs, work part-time, and have lower-paying employment [30]. Unfortunately, those who experience barriers in employment have increased challenges in caring for their children, as unemployment frequently leads to material and social deprivation. These conditions extend the period of deprivation and disadvantage for children, and as a result, further adversely impact children's developmental and health outcomes [31].

2.2.3. Education

Children being displaced and the corresponding loss of education has perhaps the most significant impact when considering human capital. For example, as of 2012, one of the greatest losses in human capital in Syria results from a loss of education, estimated at just under 11 billion US dollars, equivalent to approximately 18% of Syria's 2010 gross domestic product [32]. The right to education and its importance is emphasised in a number of international treaties, agreements, and universal goals (e.g., the United Nations Sustainable Development Goals and the *CRC*). Although primary education is critical for development, countless children are denied this right in refugee camps or in the cities of the country to which they have fled. About 7.4 million refugee and asylum-seeking children are considered under the United Nations High Commissioner for Refugees (UNHCR) as school aged. In 2017, only 61% and 23% of refugee children were enrolled in primary and secondary education, respectively, compared to 92% and 84% of children globally [33].

Low-income countries have the highest proportions of school-aged refugee and asylum-seeking children who are not in school due to limited resources and a disproportionate influx of these children to their countries compared to developed countries [34]. There are also gender inequities, where girls must overcome significant barriers to access education. Girls are often required to assist with domestic activities, such as collecting water and preparing meals, and must provide care for younger siblings and relatives. Families living in poverty may require daughters to marry young in exchange for goods or to reduce the number of children requiring care, even in the country of resettlement. Sanitation, access to private toilets and menstrual hygiene products, and the stigma around menstruation often forces girls to miss schooling. Overall, significant social and cultural barriers, as well as gender-based discrimination, threaten girls' ability to fulfil their right to education [35]. Therefore, host countries must ensure that all refugee and asylum-seeking children, regardless of their gender, receive quality education that is taught by a trained teacher following a formal curriculum [34].

Educational delays have lasting consequences on literacy, academic achievement, employment opportunity, and future socioeconomic status [31]. The quality of education is limited by the availability of resources, trained teachers, school materials, and appropriate infrastructure [36]. These limitations also affect a child's ability to receive secondary and post-secondary education, resulting in only 1% of refugee children going to university compared to 34% of people globally [34]. Benefits from education must be assessed well beyond mere academic achievement. Formal education also provides a sense of normalcy and routine, something that is often lost in the lives of refugee and asylum-seeking children. It can also improve the mental health and development of the child and provide opportunity to contribute to society and achieve goals [22,34]. Women who are educated are better prepared to care for their families, have improved health outcomes, learn independence, have fewer children, and develop leadership skills [33].

Optimal outcomes are experienced when refugee children are included and integrated in the host country's mainstream education system rather than in segregated learning environments [34]. The right to inclusive education settings guaranteed to disabled children under Article 24 of the *Convention on the Rights of Persons with Disabilities* is extended to all children, including refugee and asylum-seeking children, under the *CRC* through the joint application of Articles 2, 22, 28 and 29 [37,38]. This equal opportunity standard in education places these children on a level playing field with their peers and also accelerates their integration into their host culture [22]. Last but not least, the literature on school and community-based interventions aimed at reducing psychological disorders in refugee and asylum-seeking children indicates that interventions delivered at the school setting can successfully support children in overcoming a great deal of the difficulties associated with forced migration [39].

2.2.4. Acculturation

In their new home, refugee and asylum-seeking children must learn the host country's language and culture and begin social integration [22]. This adaptation to an unfamiliar culture is gradual and experiences such as marginalization, discrimination, bullying, xenophobia, and acculturation problems are proven harmful for the self-esteem, identity formation, and overall well-being of the child [6,22,40]. Integration into society can be an ongoing process, and participation can be limited by language barriers, cultural differences, and a lack of cultural competencies among professionals and the general public [40].

The CRC not only recognizes childhood as a critical state of growth and development, it also underlines the particular vulnerability of refugee children and asylum-seeking children due to all of the shortfalls outlined above. Therefore, to provide special measures of protection and safeguard the development of these children, it puts forth Article 22 and obligates the SPs to uphold these provisions. The following section provides an analysis of this article and presents the main attributes and themes that can assist with monitoring the implementation of Article 22.

3. Rights of Refugee and Asylum-Seeking Children under the CRC

Article 22 of the CRC obligates all SPs to " ... take appropriate measures to ensure that a child who is seeking refugee status or who is considered a refugee in accordance with applicable international or domestic law and procedures shall, whether unaccompanied or accompanied by his or her parents or by any other person, receive appropriate protection and humanitarian assistance in the enjoyment of applicable rights set forth in the present Convention and in other international human rights or humanitarian instruments to which the said States are Parties" (p.6) [1].

The preparation of Article 22, during the course of CRC drafting, took place at a time when international law first started to differentiate refugee children from adult refugees [41]. Therefore, the provision under this article captures the broad international consensus that (i) refugee children are owed appropriate protection and international assistance, (ii) all of their rights under the CRC as well as other international human rights treaties and humanitarian law must be upheld, (iii) SPs must cooperate with the UN and related agencies in order to protect and assist such children, and (iv) family reunification is a priority obligation of governments serving the best interests of children, having particular regard for unaccompanied and separated children.

3.1. The General Principles of the CRC

The principle of non-discrimination (Article 2) and its violations may often be the factor forcing children and their parents to leave their homes in search for safety. Discrimination can happen on a variety of bases, such as ethnicity, religious affiliation, or sexual orientation. Additionally, the mere designation of these children as refugees and asylum-seeking children creates a possible disadvantage and calls for the protection of Article 2 [18]. Within their new home, when these children also belong to groups like minorities, LBGTQ2, or child soldiers, they become further vulnerable. SPs must take positive measures to safeguard de facto equality for children entering their jurisdiction, as well as those children returned to their country of origin [37].

The principle of the best interests of the child (Article 3) should always remain the overarching consideration in implementation of child refugee claims under Article 22 [42]. This principle ought to be respected during all stages of the displacement cycle and decisions at any of these stages, must be appropriately documented through a formal and thorough best interest determination (BID) for each child [18,37,43].

The principle of the child's right to maximum survival and development (Article 6) and violations to this right are also, more often than not, a root causes of migration [42]. When children leave their country of origin, the protection of child rights becomes even weaker when the journeys become life threatening and high risk [41,44,45]. The SPs are obligated to take special measures to protect children by any means, for instance, through immigration policies facilitating and regulating mobility rights and not repressive detention and deportation practices, in order to protect Article 6 rights [37]. The child's right to optimal development also must inform Article 22 rights in relation to the immigration policies on the deportation or detention of a child's parent and/or guardian [37].

Lastly, under the principle of respect for the views of the child (Article 12), SPs must ensure child participation in immigration matters affecting both children and their parents. The child's best interests will play a role in both instances and children often have "their own migration projects and migration-driving factors" (pp. 9–10) [37]. Children should not be perceived as mere dependents of adult refugees and asylum-seekers; their right under Article 12 must be upheld, ensuring that their views can be expressed freely and given due consideration in relation to their age and maturity. The Committee in its General Comment (GC) No. 22 (the joint GC with the Committee on the Protection of the Rights of All Migrant Workers and Members of Their Families (CMW)) strongly reinforces these as States' Obligations [37].

The relevance of these four principles to Article 22 becomes clearer when the article is unpacked into its main attributes.

3.2. The Main Attributes of Article 22

A number of attributes were identified for each substantive right of the child under the CRC [46,47]. These attributes were determined through an exhaustive and critical appraisal of the legal standards within the major guiding documents of the CRC (these documents include, but are not limited to, relevant General Comments in the CRC and/or other human rights treaties, relevant articles and provisions under the other human rights instruments, the two *International Covenants on Civil and Political Rights* and on *Economic, Social and Cultural Rights*, relevant sections of Travaux Preparatoires, relevant CRC Concluding Observations, and the UNICEF Implementation Handbook) [47]. The attributes were identified for each CRC right in order to make its normative content concrete and to assist with the task of identifying the relevant indicators to monitor that right. In general, through this thorough analysis of relevant documents, the attributes should be able to present the essence and standards of its corresponding right [48]. Four attributes have been identified for Article 22 of the CRC, and below is a full discussion of these attributes as a result of the comprehensive analysis and appraisal.

3.2.1. Appropriate Protection and Humanitarian Assistance

Under this article, refugee and asylum-seeking children are neither granted a special status nor any lesser status than children of the host country. They are to be treated as children first and foremost and not as migrants per se, and national immigration policy cannot undermine their rights to education, health, protection, etc., under the CRC [42]. The criterion of humanitarian assistance strengthens the notion of "appropriate protection"; for example, these children may require therapy to assist with their recovery from traumatic journeys and successful integration into a new host culture [49,50]. Humanitarian assistance should avoid discriminatory consequences such as differential treatment between categories of entrants in family reunification cases [51], prohibit detention of children and possibly their parents for immigration purposes [18,42], help defend the principle of non-deportation of children [42], and reinforce the child's right to preserve family life [18,42].

3.2.2. Preservation of Rights

As a general rule, articulated under Article 2, all CRC rights apply to all children in every situation, regardless of their background. This general rule governs Article 22 as well, where refugee and asylum-seeking children are entitled to the exact same rights as any other child [1]. Article 22 refrains from reiterating all child rights one by one and rather ensures that refugee and asylum-seeking children preserve both their CRC rights and uphold the provisions and protection of other international human rights or humanitarian instruments binding on the relevant SP. Such documents provide much more extensive guidelines for SPs as to how these children are to be protected and describes, in further detail, each right and responsibility. For example, the *Inter-Agency Guiding Principles on Unaccompanied and Separated Children* are especially helpful in clarifying priority focus areas for intervening effectively with this group of particularly vulnerable children, although they should not be interpreted as minimum standards or used to read down any of the rights of unaccompanied minors under the CRC [52].

3.2.3. Duty to Protect and Assist through International Cooperation

While governments are the primary duty bearers, all parts of society can play a part in supporting the implementation of children's Article 22 rights by coming forward. For instance, provision of the right information at the right time can be critical in tracing family members and family reunification. The obligation to protect also contains a clear instruction for all duty bearers to provide children with appropriate due process—processes that do not infringe their rights to be heard and to participate in decision-making that impacts them. Such processes may require providing children with interpreters, a free legal representative, and other means in order to facilitate their meaningful participation. All the processes must be conducted in a child-friendly manner [41]. All professionals involved must be trained in child rights and be familiar with work in culturally sensitive multidisciplinary teams, including psychologists, social workers, and trauma-informed care providers, to name a few [42].

3.2.4. Best Interests and Family Reunification Principles

Two basic principles should guide every activity related to the refugee and asylum-seeking children: the principle of the best interests of the child and the principle of family unity [41]. After extensive field-testing, UNHCR adopted, in May 2008, its *Guidelines on Determining the Best Interests of the Child* [43].

As for family reunification, it should be based on a robust assessment that upholds the child's best interest as the primary consideration. Family reunification should not be delayed because of a BID procedure; however, it also cannot trump the child's best interests and would minimally require a sustainable reintegration plan avoiding any harm to the child in the country of reunification (the non-refoulement principle) and insisting upon the child's opportunity to participate in the process [18,43]. BID procedure requires a holistic child rights-based approach that considers human and financial resources, training in children's rights and inter-institutional coordination, drawing upon the cooperation and evidence available from countries of origin, transit, and destination [43].

4. Meeting the Provisions of Article 22

In relation to the four attributes of Article 22 described above, in general, countries are struggling to mitigate the effects of displacement and are failing to uphold their international commitments under Article 22 of the CRC. Within the context of developed countries, tracking these children is still a challenge, not due to the lack of resources but as a result of inadequate data collection systems that hinder the task of monitoring [53]. The section below presents some examples of SPs' efforts (or lack thereof) in meeting the provisions of Article 22 and how some States mitigate various challenges, reviewed under all four attributes discussed above.

4.1. Appropriate Protection and Humanitarian Assistance

According to this attribute, refugee and asylum-seeking children are not to be granted a special status, nor to be treated as having any lesser status than children of the host country. Therefore, children, regardless of their migration status should continue to realise all their CRC rights, including non-discriminatory access to early childhood education, formal and non-formal learning settings, and vocational and technical training. Countries such as Lebanon, Cameroon, and Uganda have strongly established inclusion of refugees in their national school systems in camp or community schools [34]. However, many countries are still struggling to uphold these commitments, such as Kenya, Pakistan, and Malaysia, where only half of the refugee population has access to primary education [34].

Many countries have already implemented legislative commitments and incentives that further reinforce provision of these rights. For example, in Canada, according to Section 30(2) of the Immigration and Refugee Protection Act (IRPA), all children who have yet to receive their immigration status, unless a temporary resident is specifically unauthorized, are automatically eligible without a permit to attend primary and secondary State schools [54]. Once the child becomes a permanent resident of Canada, attendance to public schools is mandatory [55]. Turkey also takes a similar approach to integration, despite hosting the highest number of refugees globally, most of whom are from Syria, and more than 1.7 million of whom are children [56]. Approximately 96% of registered refugees under temporary protection live in urban settings and 80% of children attend Turkish public schools. However, there is still a proportion of children not enrolled in public schools, and many secondary level students who drop out [57]. The Turkish government also runs a Conditional Cash Transfer for Education (CCTE) program in which parents receive financial incentives for each child they send to school. A particular focus is on educating girls, where the incentive is higher [56–58].

Refugee and asylum-seeking children should be treated first and foremost as children, although many immigration policies undermine their rights. As the CRC Committee states, "detention is never in the best interest of the child"; however, over 100 countries are known to detain children on the basis of their migration status [5,18]. Data regarding the exact countries and number of affected children are unknown, although there is an overall lack of child-friendly accommodations for refugee and asylum-seeking children and their families. Due to the lack of harmonized language surrounding policies for detaining children, many countries mislead and mask their regulations. As the Global Detention Project highlights, countries such as France, Poland, and Spain, amongst many others, state that children "accompany" their parents in detention centers, whereas in Canada, children are "housed as guest" with their parents. This ambiguous language around detention limits the child's ability to be recognized by the law and further prevents them from claiming their CRC rights [59].

Some countries experience a huge influx of refugees and asylum-seekers and are unable to uphold their international commitments. For instance, despite Greece's ratification of the CRC, efforts to mitigate the refugee crisis has led to controversial detention practices, many of which are a product of pressure from the European Union (EU). Many children are housed in detention centers or police stations for periods far exceeding the law of a 45-day maximum. Furthermore, many asylum-seekers are trapped in Aegean Island camps where they are subjected to a lack of food, health services, and legal representatives [60]. Turkey continues to serve as a transit country for many unregistered refugee and asylum-seekers looking to seek protection in the EU. However, due to the EU-Turkey safe-third country agreement, Greece refuses to process asylum claims or transfer refugees and asylum-seekers to the mainland, limiting the number of individuals who can enter Europe [57]. Rather, these islands act as secured facilities to process border procedures and send individuals back to Turkey, which can take months to a few years [60].

Children are frequently detained as a step towards deportation, although this often goes against the principles of non-refoulement, non-deportation, and the child's right to preserve family life [37]. If a child is to be returned, proper reintegration and reunification is essential for the child's physical and psychosocial recovery; however, such arrangements are seldom assured. In 2016, 85% of unaccompanied asylum-seeking children from Central America were apprehended in Mexico and returned to their country of origin [5].

4.2. Preservation of Rights

Unlike the almost unanimous ratification of the CRC, other international human rights treaties or humanitarian instruments do not have a high degree of ratification and support from UN member states. Many countries have yet to ratify the *1951 Convention Relating to the Status of Refugees* (Refugee Convention) or the *1967 Protocol Relation to the Status of Refugees*, the vital conventions that grant refugee and asylum-seekers necessary protection [61]. For example, only 146 SPs have ratified the Refugee Convention, where countries such as India, Bangladesh, Libya, Jordan, Nepal, Lebanon, Saudi Arabia (some of which are hosts of refugees and asylum-seekers) are among the non-ratifying countries. Conventions such as these provide much more in-depth provision for the rights of refugee and asylum-seekers and go into further details about SP responsibilities than what is described in Article 22 of the CRC [61].

Other strategies and frameworks have been adopted to strengthen the multilateralism of SPs and mitigate the increased migration between borders. Although it is not legally binding, 181 countries voted in favour (Hungary and the United States opposed the compact, and Dominican Republic, Eritrea, and Libya abstained their vote) of the *2018 Global Compact on Refugees* (compact) [62]. The *2016 New York Declaration for Refugees and Migrants* also received unprecedented support, where 193 SPs of the United Nations agreed that countries need to provide shelter and care in a more equitable, predictable, and responsible manner to refugees and asylum-seekers [63]. This demonstrates the outstanding support and intention of the global community to work collaboratively to protect the health and well-being of this vulnerable and growing population [62]. The desire to preserve rights is evident, although significant action is needed to keep SPs accountable and to uphold commitments made under international treaties, including the CRC.

4.3. Duty to Protect and Assist through International Cooperation

In general, SPs are struggling to manage safe migration of children due to insufficient resources, capacity, and political will. Lengthy and difficult processes for rendering appropriate permits, visas, and documentation, and bans on migration create significant barriers that put children in danger [5]. Professionals who interact with refugee and asylum-seeking children need to be trained in child rights, but this is rarely the case.

Research indicates that even in countries such as Denmark, Finland, Iceland, Norway, and Sweden, many border guards and police officers do not have the necessary competencies to deal with these children in a rights-based manner. There is an imbalance in the ways in which refugee and asylum-seeking children's rights are upheld and a lower standard is tolerated compared to the host country's children [64]. Often, interpreters and border security officials are not trained in child-friendly communication, which negatively influences initial contact of the children with State representatives. Finland, Norway, and Sweden provide State officials with training for identifying children who may be victims of trafficking, and protocols require the immediate contact of child protection services for unaccompanied refugee and asylum-seeking children [64].

On the positive side, the Nordic countries' child protection services adopted an interdisciplinary child-friendly approach that aims to reduce the number of interviews and conducts them in an age-appropriate manner. Information is shared among relevant central governing bodies and responsibilities are then allocated to local authorities. This has been proven to reduce levels of anxiety and mitigate the effects of trauma. However, there are many reported cases of long processing periods and miscommunication between agencies which result in a lack of services and care for children [64].

Despite efforts to provide child-friendly services and access to legal support, many children in Denmark report having inadequate information for decision-making, a problem that is particularly problematic for unaccompanied children [65]. Unaccompanied children in Sweden, Finland, and Norway have access to a guardian that represents and supports them during the legal process, although there are variations in the quality of representatives and there are often few complaint mechanisms in place for children [64,66,67].

4.4. Best Interests and Family Reunification Principles

An alarming number of refugee and asylum-seeking children leave home unaccompanied by their parents or guardians or are separated from them during the period of being on the move. There are certain regions with a disproportionate number of unaccompanied children traveling alone, such as through the Central Mediterranean route. This route is not only one of the most dangerous and deadly migration channels (1 in 40 rate of mortality) but it is also a highly common route used for unaccompanied and separated children. In 2017, unaccompanied children made up 92% of all children arriving by sea [5]. Other regions such as the United States and Mexico border are also seeing increases in such trends, whereby 100,000 unaccompanied and separated children were apprehended in 2015–2016 [5].

Most countries contain a number of different legal barriers within their policies and procedures that create difficulties for family reunification and thus "prevent many children from enjoying the right to respect and enjoyment of the family life to which they are entitled" (p. 33) [68]. For instance, in certain circumstances, parents who migrated before their children have limited legal means for reunification. Long waiting periods lasting two to three years, insufficient income, age limitations, and restrictions for de facto dependent reunification all prolong periods of separation from loved ones [68]. In the United States for example, "children granted the Special Immigration Juvenile Status, a visa created to provide a permanent legal status for children found to have been 'abused, abandoned or neglected' can never exercise family reunion rights" (p.5) [69]. In order to be reunited with family, the child must reach adulthood and prove that their parents are dependent on them [69].

There are also significant economic limitations that create barriers for family reunification. Canada and Turkey both have shown good faith to the principle of family reunification; however, even in these countries, the applicants must satisfy a number of criteria to be eligible. For instance, the family member seeking reunification must be able to sponsor the spouse and/or dependent child(ren), demonstrate that they are financially capable of supporting their loved one(s) in the host country, and satisfy regulations of self-sufficiency [70,71]. Alternatively, in Canada, private sponsorship programs are available to help support reunification, although this is reliant on a Canadian citizen or group to fully financially support the individual or family moving to Canada [72]. Furthermore, the initial application claim must indicate all dependents to be eligible for reunification. This creates barriers as many may not be able to meet these requirements or may only be able to sponsor a few family members. Consequently, a spouse and/or the remaining children may be left behind, waiting the lengthy administrative process for the decision of their claim, or until the family is financially capable to support them. Countries can also create barriers by declaring a country in which a family member resides as 'safe', deeming them ineligible to apply for asylum and requiring them to follow the lengthy immigration processes instead [5].

There are, however, programs for family reunification that assist vulnerable families fleeing their country of origin. For example, the International Organization for Migration's Family Assistance Program provides reunification services for individuals with a protection status in Germany. There are service centers in ten countries, including Turkey, Lebanon, and Iraq, that provide safe reunification services, facilitate visa processing and meetings with the countries' Consulates, and empower families through preservation of rights. Services are provided in their preferred language, and facilities are accessible for individuals with disabilities, as well as designed to be family and child-friendly [73]. For the Canadian resettlement sponsorship applications, determining whether a young child "for whom the family has been caring and whose parents have been killed or are missing" can be considered a de facto dependent and aligns with *CRC* principles. All decisions must be conducted with the child's best interest in mind and officials must ensure there are no disputes with guardianship. Before finalizing any cases, Canadian officers must ensure that the UNHCR conducted a BID assessment for the child's referral [74].

5. Conclusions

This paper presents just a glimpse into the current global climate for refugee and asylum-seeking children. One area of these children's lives that is increasingly and rightfully gaining attention is ensuring that children are receiving quality and equitable opportunities for education. There is also more support and acknowledgement from the global community expressing the urgency and commitment to protect child rights and improve the overall conditions of these children, as indicated, for example, by the *Global Compact on Refugees* and the *New York Declaration for Refugees and Migrants* [62,63]. However, it is time to move past expressing the desire to support these individuals and rather work towards implementing the necessary structural and procedural commitments to ensure rights are being preserved.

There is still much to learn about safeguarding migration channels and ensuring that risks are mitigated as children move across borders. Many of the detrimental ramifications on health and development, such as trauma, being separated from loved ones, and exploitation, are exacerbated by the dangerous journeys to safety. At the landing point, globally, there is a need for more child-friendly accommodations and services, especially for children waiting for claims to be processed. During this period of uncertainty and fear, many children are housed with parents in adult facilities and are prevented from claiming other CRC rights, such as education, health, and play. In particular, during these periods, unaccompanied refugee and asylum-seeking children need access to all the information that concerns them and must be provided appropriate legal representation, although we see that this is often not the case in areas such as Central America [5]. As discussed above, there are many existing barriers preventing expedited family reunification processes, further prolonging periods of separation and affecting all domains of health.

At a national level, there needs to be better accountability, monitoring, and reporting mechanisms in place to ensure that SPs are upholding their CRC and other international commitments.

Collecting timely and accurate data regarding the provision of rights for refugee and asylum-seeking children is necessary to ensure that SPs are accountable for maintaining both their national and international obligations under the CRC. The SPs, in accordance with their obligations under the CRC in general (and Article 22 in particular) must implement structural commitments in the form of legislation and policies in support of the refugee and asylum-seeking children they host. They must make every effort to ensure that processes align with the general principles of promoting the rights of these children to life and maximum development (Article 6) in a non-discriminatory manner (Article 2). The children's best interest (Article 3) must remain at the center of their decisions while they provide children with ample opportunities to participate, voice their opinions, and to be heard during these decision-making processes (Article 12) [1]. Last but not least, the SPs must collect and periodically report disaggregated data on all the rights of refugee and asylum-seeking children.

Widespread public awareness raising is required to overcome tribulations such as xenophobia and discrimination demonstrated from the citizens which add to the difficulties faced by these children. These perceptions and behaviours of the citizens can often influence the predicament of newcomers adversely, not just by adding to the stressors in the environment but also by influencing State immigration laws and protocols in a negative manner. Consequently, added means for refusing refugees may be implemented, such as building walls, detaining individuals, closing borders, stopping boats from docking in their country, and returning individuals to their unsafe country of origin by force [5].

Pediatricians, educators, social workers, and professionals working for and/or with refugee and asylum-seeking children are best equipped to advocate for their rights. Action in this domain is two-fold: to ensure that services are conducted in a culturally safe and sensitive manner, and to ensure that the voices of these vulnerable populations are heard. By careful monitoring, reporting, and advocating for the needs of children on the move, care providers can provide a stronger voice to this often-silenced population. By partaking in discussions, joining advocacy groups, and creating safe spaces for newly resettled families, care providers have the ability to influence decision-makers and the general population.

All in all, while some countries have not yet had to deal with complex migration issues to the same degree that others have, with climate change exacerbation, increased civil unrest, and the proliferation of channels for illegal transit, the planet will be experiencing a further increase in the phenomenon of children on the move across its four corners. All countries and indeed, human societies, must come together to reduce the burden and hardship of refugee and asylum-seeking children who travel long distances, experience horrifying journeys, and all too often face discouraging outcomes prior to, during, and even after their resettlement. Working with the provisions of Article 22 while maintaining the principles the *CRC* can serve as a guide in this enormous and remarkably important task.

Author Contributions: Z.V. led the development of this manuscript, drafted several sections, and responded to review comments; Z.T. conducted the research, authored several sections, and completed revisions of all drafts; C.W. contributed to the first draft of the analysis of Article 22, and provided feedback on several drafts of the manuscript.

Funding: This manuscript was prepared relying upon the generous funds granted to Z.V. by the Michael Smith Foundation for Health Research (MSFHR) and the Canadian Institute for Health Research (CIHR).

Acknowledgments: We acknowledge and greatly appreciate the careful read through and insightful feedback of Rajvir Gill, JD, from the New Brunswick Office of Child and Youth Advocate on this paper.

Conflicts of Interest: The authors declare no conflict of interest.

References

1. Convention on the Rights of the Child. Available online: https://www.ohchr.org/en/professionalinterest/pages/crc (accessed on 15 August 2019).
2. United Nations Treaty Collection. Convention on the Rights of the Child. Available online: https://treaties.un.org/Pages/ViewDetails.aspx?src=IND&mtdsg_no=IV-11&chapter=4&lang=en (accessed on 3 October 2019).
3. Convention and Protocol Relating to the Status of Refugees. Available online: https://www.unhcr.org/3b66c2aa10.html (accessed on 17 July 2019).
4. Global Trends: Forced Displacement in 2018. Available online: https://www.unhcr.org/5d08d7ee7.pdf (accessed on 6 August 2019).
5. A Child Is a Child: Protecting Children on the Move from Violence, Abuse and Exploitation. Available online: https://data.unicef.org/resources/child-child-protecting-children-move-violence-abuse-exploitation/ (accessed on 6 August 2019).
6. International Society for Social Pediatrics and Child Health (ISSOP). ISSOP position statement on migrant child health. *Child Care Health Dev.* **2017**, *44*, 161–170.
7. Fisher, J. The four domains model: Connecting spirituality, health and well-being. *Religions* **2011**, *2*, 17–28. [CrossRef]
8. Felitti, V.J.; Anda, R.F.; Nordenberg, D.; Williamson, D.F.; Spitz, A.M.; Edwards, V.; Koss, M.P.; Marks, J.S. Relationship of childhood abuse and household dysfunction to many of the leading causes of death in adults. The Adverse Childhood Experiences (ACE) Study. *Am. J. Prev Med.* **1998**, *14*, 245–258. [CrossRef]
9. Centers for Disease Control and Prevention. About the CDC-Kaiser ACE Study. Available online: https://www.cdc.gov/violenceprevention/childabuseandneglect/acestudy/about.html (accessed on 3 October 2019).
10. Manyema, M.; Norris, S.A.; Richter, L.M. Stress begets stress: The association of adverse childhood experiences with psychological distress in the presence of adult life stress. *BMC Public Health* **2018**, *8*, 835. [CrossRef]
11. Pfeil, J.; Hufnagel, M. Rational diagnostics and therapies in child refugees. *Pediatr. Infect. Dis. J.* **2018**, *37*, 272–274. [CrossRef]
12. Riggs, E.; Rajan, S.; Casey, S.; Kilpatrick, N. Refugee child oral health. *Oral Dis.* **2017**, *23*, 292–299. [CrossRef]
13. Keygnaert, I.; Vettenburg, N.; Roelens, K.; Temmerman, M. Sexual health is dead in my body: Participatory assessment of sexual health determinants by refugees, asylum seekers and undocumented migrants in Belgium and the Netherlands. *BMC Public Health* **2014**, *14*, 416–429. [CrossRef]
14. Charania, N.; Paynter, J.; Lee, A.; Watson, D.; Turner, N. Exploring immunisation inequities among migrant and refugee children in New Zealand. *Hum. Vaccin. Immunother.* **2018**, *14*, 3026–3033. [CrossRef]
15. Williams, T.; Chopra, V.; Chikanya, S. "It isn't that we're prostitutes": Child protection and sexual exploitation of adolescent girls within and beyond refugee camps in Rwanda. *Child Abus. Negl.* **2018**, *86*, 158–166. [CrossRef]
16. Hossain, M.; Zimmerman, C.; Abas, M.; Light, M.; Watts, C. The relationship of trauma to mental disorders among trafficked and sexually exploited girls and women. *Am. J. Public Health* **2010**, *100*, 2442–2449. [CrossRef]
17. Rossiter, M.J.; Hatami, S.; Ripley, D.; Rossiter, K.R. Immigrant and refugee youth settlement experiences: "A new kind of war". *Int. J. Child Youth Fam. Stud.* **2009**, *6*, 746–770. [CrossRef]

18. United Nations Committee on the Rights of the Child. General Comment No. 6: Treatment of Unaccompanied and Separated Children outside Their Country of Origin (CRC/GC/2005/6, 2005). Available online: https://www.refworld.org/docid/42dd174b4.html (accessed on 6 August 2019).
19. Drury, J.; Williams, R. Children and young people who are refugees, internally displaced persons or survivors or perpetrators of war, mass violence and terrorism. *Curr. Opin. Psychiatry* **2012**, *25*, 277–284. [CrossRef] [PubMed]
20. Skudoor, J. Trauma and children: A refugee perspective. *Child. Aust.* **2015**, *40*, 188–194.
21. Kronick, R.; Rousseau, C.; Cleveland, J. Refugee children's sandplay narratives in immigration detention in Canada. *Eur. Child Adolesc. Psychiatry* **2017**, *27*, 423–437. [CrossRef] [PubMed]
22. Fazel, M.; Reed, R.; Panter-Brick, C.; Stein, A. Mental health of displaced and refugee children resettled in high-income countries: Risk and protective factors. *Lancet* **2012**, *379*, 266–282. [CrossRef]
23. Shonkoff, J.P. Leveraging the biology of adversity to address the roots of disparities in health and development. *Proc. Natl. Acad. Sci. USA* **2012**, *109*, 17302–17307. [CrossRef]
24. Cassidy, J.; Shaver, P.R. *Handbook of Attachment: Theory, Research, and Clinical Applications*, 2nd ed.; The Guilford Press: New York, NY, USA, 2008; pp. 12–444.
25. Hertzman, C.; Boyce, T. How experiences gets under the skin to create gradients in developmental health. *Annu. Rev. Public Health* **2010**, *31*, 329–347. [CrossRef]
26. Dalgaard, N.; Todd, B.; Daniel, S.; Montgomery, E. The transmission of trauma in refugee families: Associations between intra-family trauma communication style, children's attachment security and psychosocial adjustment. *Attach. Hum. Dev.* **2015**, *18*, 69–89. [CrossRef]
27. Carey, N. Introduction. In *The Epigenetics Revolution: How Modern Biology Is Rewriting Our Understanding of Genetics, Disease, and Inheritance*, 1st ed.; Carey, N., Ed.; Columbia University Press: New York, NY, USA, 2012; pp. 1–9.
28. Yehuda, R.; Daskalakis, N.P.; Bierer, L.M.; Bader, H.N.; Klengel, T.; Holsboer, F.; Binder, E.B. Holocaust exposure induced intergenerational effect on FKBP5 methylation. *Biol. Psychiatry* **2016**, *80*, 372–380. [CrossRef]
29. Stein, A.D.; Pierik, F.H.; Verrips, G.H.W.; Susser, E.S.; Lumey, L.H. Maternal exposure to the Dutch Famine before conception and during pregnancy: Quality of life and depressive symptoms in adult offspring. *Epidemiology* **2009**, *20*, 909–915. [CrossRef]
30. Wilkinson, L.; Garcea, J. *The Economic Integration of Refugees in Canada: A Mixed Record?* 1st ed.; Migration Policy Institute: Washington, DC, USA, 2017; pp. 9–12.
31. Social Determinants of Health: The Canadian Facts. Available online: http://thecanadianfacts.org/The_Canadian_Facts.pdf (accessed on 17 July 2019).
32. Economic Loss from School Dropout Due to the Syria Crisis. Available online: http://wos-education.org/uploads/reports/Economic_loss_study_English_FINAL.pdf (accessed on 9 October 2019).
33. Turn the Tide: Refugee Education in Crisis. Available online: https://www.unhcr.org/5b852f8e4.pdf (accessed on 17 July 2019).
34. Missing out: Refugee Education in Crisis. UNHCR Education Report. 2016. Available online: https://www.unhcr.org/57d9d01d0 (accessed on 31 July 2019).
35. Her Turn. It's Time to Make Refugee Girls' Education a Priority. Available online: https://www.unhcr.org/herturn/ (accessed on 3 October 2019).
36. Education Uprooted: For Every Migrant, Refugee and Displaced Child, Education. Available online: https://www.unicef.org/publications/files/UNICEF_Education_Uprooted.pdf (accessed on 8 August 2019).
37. Joint General Comment No. 3 (2017) of the Committee on the Protection of the Rights of All Migrant Workers and Members of Their Families and No. 22 (2017) of the Committee on the Rights of the Child on the General Principles Regarding the Human Rights of Children in the Context of International Migration (CMW/C/GC/3-CRC/C/GC/22, 2017). Available online: https://www.refworld.org/docid/5a1293a24.html (accessed on 7 August 2019).
38. Joint General Comment No. 4 (2017) of the Committee on the Protection of the Rights of All Migrant Workers and Members of Their Families and No. 23 (2017) of the Committee on the Rights of the Child on State Obligations Regarding the Human Rights of Children in the Context of International Migration in Countries of Origin, Transit, Destination and Return* (CMW/C/GC/4-CRC/C/GC/23, 2017). Available online: https://www.refworld.org/docid/5a12942a2b.html (accessed on 8 August 2019).

39. Tyrer, R.A.; Fazel, M. School and community-based interventions for refugee and asylum seeking children: A systematic review. *PLoS ONE* **2014**, *9*, e97977. [CrossRef] [PubMed]
40. Edge, S.; Newbold, B. Discrimination and the health of immigrants and refugees: Exploring Canada's evidence base and directions for future research in newcomer receiving countries. *J. Immigr. Minor. Health* **2012**, *15*, 141–148. [CrossRef] [PubMed]
41. Vuckovic Sahovic, N.; Doek, J.; Zermatten, J. Notification to Executive Committee on Refugee Children. In *The Rights of the Child in International Law*, 1st ed.; Vuckovic Sahovic, N., Doek, J., Zermatten, J., Eds.; Stämpfli Publishers: Berne, Switzerland, 2012; pp. 231–232.
42. Ceriani Cemadas, P. The human rights of children in the context of international migration. In *Routledge International Handbook of Children's Rights Studies*, 1st ed.; Vandenhole, W., Desmet, E., Reynaert, D., Lembrechts, S., Eds.; Routledge: London, UK; New York, NY, USA, 2015; pp. 331–357.
43. *UNHCR Guidelines on Determining the Best Interests of the Child*; UN High Commission for Refugees (UNHCR): Geneva, Switzerland, 2008; pp. 1–100. Available online: https://www.unhcr.org/4566b16b2.pdf (accessed on 26 July 2019).
44. Van Bueren, G. *Child Rights in Europe: Convergence and Divergence in Judicial Protection*, 1st ed.; Council of Europe Publishing: Strasbourg, France, 2007; p. 123.
45. Harris, D.; O'Boyle, M.; Buckley, C. *Law of the European Convention on Human Rights*, 2nd ed.; Oxford University Press: Oxford, UK, 2009.
46. Vaghri, Z.; Krappmann, L.; Doek, J. From the Indicators of General Comment 7 to GlobalChild: A Decade of Work to Enhance Accountability to Children. *Int. J. Child. Rights* **2019**, *27*, 1–31, in press.
47. Vaghri, Z.; Zermatten, J.; Lansdown, G.; Ruggiero, R. Unpacking the Substantive Rights of Children under the Convention on the Rights of the Child. In Preparation.
48. Human Rights Indicators: A Guide to Measurement and Implementation. Available online: https://www.ohchr.org/Documents/Publications/Human_rights_indicators_en.pdf (accessed on 6 August 2019).
49. UNICEF. *Implementation Handbook for the Convention on the Rights of the Child: Fully Revised Third Edition*; United Nations Publications: Geneva, Switzerland, 2007; p. 306.
50. Considerations of Reports Submitted by States Parties under Article 44 of the Convention: Concluding Observations: Norway (CRC/C/15/Add.263, 2015) (para. 42). Available online: https://www.refworld.org/docid/45377ea20.html (accessed on 6 August 2019).
51. Considerations of Reports Submitted by States Parties under Article 44 of the Convention: Concluding Observations: Australia (CRC/C/15/Add.268, 2015). Available online: https://www.refworld.org/docid/45377eac0.html (accessed on 7 August 2019).
52. *Inter-Agency Guiding Principles on Unaccompanied and Separated Children*; International Committee of the Red Cross: Geneva, Switzerland, 2004; Available online: https://www.unicef.org/protection/IAG_UASCs.pdf (accessed on 7 August 2019).
53. A Call to Action: Protecting Children on the Move Starts with Better Data. Available online: https://data.unicef.org/resources/call-action-protecting-children-move-starts-better-data/ (accessed on 25 July 2019).
54. Immigrant and Refugee Protection Act. Available online: https://laws-lois.justice.gc.ca/eng/acts/i-2.5/FullText.html (accessed on 25 July 2019).
55. UNHCR Resettlement Handbook—Canada Chapter. Available online: https://www.unhcr.org/3c5e55594.pdf (accessed on 25 July 2019).
56. UNHCR Turkey Fact Sheet. Available online: https://reliefweb.int/sites/reliefweb.int/files/resources/01.-UNHCR-Turkey-Fact-Sheet-August-2018.pdf (accessed on 25 August 2019).
57. UNICEF Turkey 2018 Humanitarian Results. Available online: https://reliefweb.int/sites/reliefweb.int/files/resources/UNICEF%20Turkey%20Humanitarian%20Situation%20Report%20No.%2028%20-%20January-December%202018.pdf (accessed on 26 July 2019).
58. Syria Crisis Humanitarian Relief Operation. Available online: https://www.kizilay.org.tr/Upload/Dokuman/Dosya/april-019-syria-crisis-humanitarian-relief-operation-24-05-2019-06655246.pdf (accessed on 31 July 2019).
59. Global Detention Project Annual Report. 2018. Available online: https://www.globaldetentionproject.org/global-detention-project-annual-report-2018 (accessed on 4 October 2019).
60. Greece: Stranded in Aegean Limbo. Available online: https://www.globaldetentionproject.org/greece-stranded-in-aegean-limbo (accessed on 4 October 2019).

61. United Nations Treaty Collection, Convention Relating to the Status of Refugees. Available online: https://treaties.un.org/pages/ViewDetailsII.aspx?src=TREATY&mtdsg_no=V-2&chapter=5&Temp=mtdsg2&clang=_en (accessed on 7 October 2019).
62. UN Affirms 'Historic' Global Compact to Support World's Refugees. Available online: https://news.un.org/en/story/2018/12/1028791 (accessed on 7 October 2019).
63. What Is the Global Compact on Refugees? Available online: https://www.unhcr.org/ph/the-global-compact-on-refugees (accessed on 8 October 2019).
64. Protected on Paper? An Analysis of Nordic Country Response to Asylum-Seeking Children. UNICEF Office of Research-Innocenti. Available online: https://www.unicef-irc.org/publications/pdf/NORDIC%2028%20LOWRES.pdf (accessed on 7 October 2019).
65. Concluding Observations on the Fifth Periodic Report of Denmark (CRC/C/DNK/CO/5). Available online: https://www.refworld.org/publisher,CRC,CONCOBSERVATIONS,DNK,5a0ebb974,0.html (accessed on 9 October 2019).
66. Concluding Observations on the Fifth Periodic Report of Sweden (CRC/C/SWE/CO/5). Available online: https://www.refworld.org/type,CONCOBSERVATIONS,,SWE,566e7e8c4,0.html (accessed on 9 October 2019).
67. Concluding Observations on the Twenty-Fifth Periodic Report of Finland (CERD/C/FIN/CO/23). Available online: https://www.refworld.org/type,CONCOBSERVATIONS,,FIN,5978a4114,0.html (accessed on 9 October 2019).
68. Bhabha, J. *Child Migration & Human Rights in a Global Age*, 1st ed.; Princeton University Press: Princeton, NJ, USA, 2014; pp. 20–33.
69. Bhabha, J. *Independent Children, Inconsistent Adults: International Child Migration and the Legal Framework*; Innocenti Discussion Paper No. IDP2008 02; UNICEF Innocenti Research Centre: Florence, Italy, 2008.
70. Sponsor Your Spouse, Partner or Child: About the Process. Available online: https://www.canada.ca/en/immigration-refugees-citizenship/services/immigrate-canada/family-sponsorship/spouse-partner-children.html (accessed on 17 July 2019).
71. Turkey: Law No. 6458 of 2013 on Foreigners and International Protection (as amended 29 Oct 2016). Available online: https://www.refworld.org/docid/5a1d828f4.html (accessed on 7 August 2019).
72. Sponsor a Refugee. Available online: https://www.canada.ca/en/immigration-refugees-citizenship/services/refugees/help-outside-canada/private-sponsorship-program.html (accessed on 16 July 2019).
73. International Organization for Migration: Family Reunification. Available online: https://turkey.iom.int/family-reunification (accessed on 7 October 2019).
74. Processing Family Members as Part of a Resettlement Sponsorship Application. Available online: https://www.canada.ca/en/immigration-refugees-citizenship/corporate/publications-manuals/operational-bulletins-manuals/refugee-protection/resettlement/eligibility/determining-which-family-members-eligible-resettlement.html (accessed on 9 October 2019).

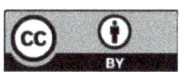

© 2019 by the authors. Licensee MDPI, Basel, Switzerland. This article is an open access article distributed under the terms and conditions of the Creative Commons Attribution (CC BY) license (http://creativecommons.org/licenses/by/4.0/).

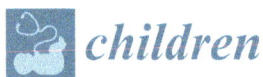

Brief Report

Gender-Related Challenges in Educational Interventions with Syrian Refugee Parents of Trauma-Affected Children in Turkey

Melissa Diamond [1] and Charles Oberg [2],*

1. A Global Voice for Autism, Minneapolis, MN 55442, USA; melissa@aglobalvoiceforautism.org
2. Division of Global Pediatrics, University of Minnesota, MN 55415, USA
* Correspondence: oberg001@umn.edu

Received: 20 August 2019; Accepted: 19 September 2019; Published: 7 October 2019

Abstract: Since 2012, more than three million Syrian refugees have fled to Turkey. While these refugees vary in socioeconomic background, it is notable that 50% of Syrian refugee children in Turkey display symptoms of post-traumatic stress and that more than 663,138 of these children between the ages of six and seventeen are not enrolled in school. For those children who are in school, high levels of trauma have significant implications for the education system as trauma alters the brain and affects the way children learn. A Global Voice for Autism is an international non-governmental relief and development organization that exists to equip teachers and families in conflict-affected communities. Its intent is to support the development and success of children with autism and trauma-related behavioral challenges in their classrooms, home, and communities. The instabilities inherent in the Syrian refugee experience pose a number of challenges to the organization's effective implementation of programming. The experiences of refugees in Turkey are highly gendered. Therefore, a qualitative gender analysis was conducted to address and better understand the challenges faced when carrying out these educational interventions. The article examines domestic violence, sexual violence, and masculinity as gender-driven constructs that influence how refugees experience trauma. In addition, structural issues in existing support systems all present significant challenges to Syrian refugee parents that impede effective program implementation. It is imperative to assess structural issues in existing support services to address these challenges and to successfully carry out meaningful and impactful programming. This Brief Report provides a series of recommendations in order to ameliorate these challenges and increase the efficacy of educational interventions with Syrian refugee parents of trauma-affected and vulnerable children in Turkey. It concludes with a call for policy changes that protect refugees from deportation when accessing support services and a network of services that do not require residency permits. It calls for increased integration of parent trauma support in educational intervention trainings and the creation of safe spaces where mothers and fathers can discuss their own trauma and challenges in the hope of significantly enhancing program efficacy.

Keywords: refugee; gender; trauma; educational intervention

1. Introduction

Since 2012, more than three million Syrian refugees have fled to Turkey. While these refugees vary in socioeconomic background, it is notable that 50% of Syrian refugee children in Turkey display symptoms of post-traumatic stress [1]. A significant number of these children are not in school and for those children who are in school, high levels of trauma have significant implications for the education system as trauma alters the brain and affects the way children learn.

Syrian refugees in Turkey have tended to settle in concentrated communities. This has some advantages for Syrians who, for the most part, do not speak Turkish and whose cultural differences pose challenges, particularly within the education system. Across Turkey, an estimated 663,138 refugee children between the ages of six and seventeen are not enrolled in school [2]. Until recently, many Syrian refugees hesitated to send their children to school due to a perception that their stay in Turkey was temporary. However, as families started to realize the permanency of their residence in Turkey, school enrollment has steadily increased.

Research shows that effective education actively contributes to children's development of skills for coping and resilience, which are key skills in a population where research shows children experience post-traumatic stress. However, even when Syrian refugees are enrolled in school, their ability to access an inclusive and effective education is limited. Overcrowding in the schools and a lack of trained teachers pose challenges to the education system. Furthermore, unsupportive or unstable home environments can interfere with the quality of a child's education [3]. These challenges have a particular impact on trauma-affected children, who learn differently due to brain changes triggered by trauma, and children with learning differences such as Autism Spectrum Disorder [4]. The effects of trauma on learning are influenced by the regulation of hormones, particularly cortisol and neurotransmitters in response to stress leading to a state of chronic persistent arousal. This triggers a "fight or flight" reflex that interferes with learning and the acquisition of new knowledge. This helps to explain how stress within the context of the learning experience, regardless of the cause of that stress, can result in alteration in attention, memory and other learning processes [5,6].

2. Gender and the Nature of Trauma

Refugees by definition are persons who have fled their country of origin for reasons of feared persecution, war, conflict, or generalized violence and, as a result, require protection [7]. Many have suffered trauma, with a residual impact on their health and well-being [8]. By virtue of the ways that men and women have different refugee experiences, displaced men and women also cope with trauma in different ways. Trauma complicates and interferes with daily life regardless of gender. However, the ways in which it complicates and influences supports that are necessary differ for men and women due to perceptions about the gendered needs of refugee populations. This can have dangerous implications.

For mothers, who are traditionally the primary caregivers within the Syrian population, an inability to adequately provide for their children during displacement can be traumatizing [9]. This trauma and inability to cope can result in decreased self-esteem and increased parenting stress, which inhibit mothers' abilities to implement learned educational practices at home with confidence as well as their abilities to create safe, supportive home environments for trauma-affected children. In addition, a mother may be stigmatized for having a child with a disability and/or who has experienced significant trauma. In addition, typical home-based care roles prevent the formation of social groups in Turkey [10]. This isolation can exacerbate the manifestations of parental trauma in the home, while relegation to the home leaves mothers without access to psychological support.

Experiences in the home are one of the primary contributors to traumatic stress in children [11]. Insufficient parental trauma support can destabilize a child's home environment through neglect and violence [12]. Even young children who were born in Turkey and have never experienced war in Syria are experiencing trauma as a result of the manifestations of parental trauma in their homes. Parents must have access to the support they need in order to create safe, healthy environments for their children, and such environments are crucial for the effective education of trauma-affected children.

2.1. Sexual Violence

Sexual violence has historically been used as a tool in conflict, and the Syrian conflict is no exception [13]. The use of rape as punishment in Syrian prisons has been documented, as has widespread sexual assault in refugee camps and sexual violence in the home [14]. In 2013 alone, the UN found 38,000 victims of sexual violence in Syria, including women, men, and children, despite significant underreporting.

Due to the stigma of sexual assault, emphasis on virginity, and the reality of honor killings, women hesitate to report experiences of sexual violence. For men, especially men who were once active in the Syrian conflict, sexual abuse is also a reality. The stigma of sexual violence is significant for both men and women in the community. For women, discovered incidences of sexual assault from someone other than a marital partner can lead to divorce, which is particularly threatening in a refugee context where there are fewer chances for a woman to achieve financial sustainability and support her children on her own [15]. Such discoveries may even result in honor killings [16]. For men, discovery of sexual assault can lead to community ostracism, blackmail, and loss of employment [17]. Even when not expressed or reported, these experiences can severely inhibit a caregiver's ability to offer support to the children they are teaching or raising.

Women may also experience sexual violence from their husbands. This violence may be a continuation of ongoing sexual violence from before the conflict but may also materialize as a result of men's unaddressed trauma and marginalization of masculinity in the refugee context [18]. While all sexual violence can result in trauma, sexual violence within the marital relationship may have the greatest impact on educational interventions for trauma-affected children due to the effects of ongoing sexual violence. Teachers who experience ongoing sexual violence may have less ability to concentrate on the needs of their students in the classroom, while sexual violence between parents at home alters family dynamics and can create a dangerous living environment for children. Finally, for refugee families who have lost everything, the pressure to earn money can force children into early marriage, taking them out of school and making them less likely to ever return [19].

2.2. Domestic Violence

Domestic violence occurs in a variety of ways for Syrian refugees living in Turkey. In some families, domestic violence is a continuation or a worsening of domestic violence perpetrated in Syria, while for others it is a new phenomenon. Both men and women perpetrate this violence, and children are often the victims of parental rage. Men are typically thought of as the perpetrators of domestic violence. However, women, lacking mental health support and grappling with the stresses of insecurity and isolation, often take out their frustrations on their children [20]. This creates a sense of insecurity for children at home, inhibits the efficacy of positive reinforcement approaches, and can exacerbate the trauma experienced by children [21]. Additionally, many Syrian women who flee to Turkey without husbands marry Turkish men, who often take them as second wives [22]. These situations leave women and their children vulnerable to abuse, and they are often tasked with household maintenance. Because Turkey does not recognize polygamous marriages, women in these marriages are especially vulnerable to abuse. Many Syrian women enter into these arrangements as a means of survival and cannot leave their husbands due to financial dependence [22].

One mother in A Global Voice for Autism's program reported that, when she told her parents that her husband beat her so severely that she required hospitalization, her parents had asked her what she had done to upset her husband and told her to be more obedient in the future [23]. Without safe home environments that meet their own needs, parents cannot concentrate on the needs of their children. It is notable that in all of these scenarios, there is a trend of victim blaming by the broader community, which leads to a hesitancy in reporting or seeking support [24].

Given the strong gender norms in Syrian culture, aid agencies often dismiss sexual abuse and domestic violence as cultural factors that are not within the parameters of their mandates to support displacement-related needs [25]. This view not only allows domestic violence to continue without intervention, but also results in detrimental impacts on numerous other factors, such as children's education, that aid organizations seek to address in times of conflict.

2.3. Masculinity

Historically, displacement has presented opportunities for gender roles to be renegotiated within displaced communities. Because of this, many community organizations in Turkey seek to challenge established gender roles within Syrian culture that define men as breadwinners and women as caregivers. In the camps, women are assigned leadership roles to challenge traditional gender structures. Outside of the camps, women's employment schemes aim to shift breadwinner dynamics within the household [26].

However, when focused solely on women, such interventions have detrimental effects on men that can spill over into negative consequences for wives and children. Without access to support and opportunities, men's pent-up frustrations can transform into domestic violence in an attempt to regain control amid feelings of marginalization [27]. Even without contrived shifts in gender roles, displacement challenges Syrian men's conceptions of their own masculinity. Relocation to Turkey coincides with a loss of meaningful work, demotion to refugee status, and limited opportunities to provide for a family and make personal decisions [28].

These losses are coupled with increased time spent consuming media. Unemployed and seeking connections to home, refugee men access more televised media than ever before. Much of the media consumed is related to the war and emphasizes militaristic and violent conceptions of masculinity in its portrayals of fighting. However, even international news coverage of refugees reinforces these concepts of masculinity [29]. In depicting women and children as vulnerable and innocent and men as violent and dangerous migrants, the media reinforces understandings of masculinity that link it to violence [30].

Without productive outlets such as employment, and no support in the development of new masculine identities, masculinity can manifest as violence [31]. However, even when this does not occur, traditional narratives about Syrian masculinity can discourage fathers from engaging in caregiving activities. This makes it more difficult to include fathers in educational interventions. Because the practices that A Global Voice for Autism uses emphasize consistency, fathers' lack of engagement can lead them to act in ways that counteract efforts to support their children's learning using evidence-based practices [32].

2.4. Qualitative Gender Analysis

In order to understand and address the challenges that A Global Voice for Autism faces when carrying out these educational interventions, a qualitative gender analysis was conducted. Utilizing a combination of primary and secondary data, essential findings were identified related to the aforementioned barriers and their implications. Primary data was collated from A Global Voice for Autism's past programs for Syrian refugees in Turkey along with data and information from secondary sources from partner organizations, researchers, and other community actors. Data collection methods included structured and unstructured narrative interviews, surveys, indices, video analyses, incident reports, and structured observation sessions. Of those families participating in educational support programing, 23% of families experienced past or present food and shelter insecurity, 27% reported experiencing domestic violence, and 14% reported experiencing sexual violence [33].

3. Structural Issues in Existing Support Systems

Children have specific rights, as articulated in the UN Convention on the Rights of the Child [34]. It has been thirty years since its adoption by the UN General Assembly, and it is as necessary now as when it went into effect. The convention articulates the principles of protection from harm, provision of basic needs, and the active participation of children as rights holders. Specifically, Article 22 states that countries must take appropriate measures to protect and assist all families of refugee children. It is from this context that structural deficiencies in existing support systems are explored [35].

Structural issues within Turkey exacerbate the impact of trauma and domestic and sexual violence in the Syrian refugee population. Although Turkey's public hospitals offer free healthcare to residents, language barriers limit the ability of Syrian residents to access psychological support. Additionally, many public services that are theoretically available require that users hold a residency permit for their area of residence. However, the exorbitant costs of these residency permits are cost-prohibitive to most Syrian refugees, and an estimated 81% of women living outside of the camps do not hold permits [36]. Because of this, Syrians risk deportation to camps or back to Syria if they access the services that are theoretically available to address domestic and sexual violence. This is a particular vulnerability for women and children for whom the lack of privacy and threatened bodily integrity in the camp cause more immediate issues than they do for men.

In addition to the challenges that exist within the public support system, the private organizations that provide such supports to Syrians are often riddled with corruption. Family name, conflict party, and bribery all play roles in determining who has access to these services [37]. Even when people are in a social position to access these services, confidentiality is often compromised. Hence these services are not accessed due to the breech of confidence in the eyes of Syrians suffering from stigmatized experiences.

4. Components of Effective Educational Interventions

In order to address the aforementioned challenges within educational settings for Syrian refugees, A Global Voice for Autism works to equip communities with the skills and support they need to support trauma-affected children and children with autism in their classrooms, homes, and communities. Recognizing the interplay between home environment and effective education, the organization takes a holistic approach to their mission. Parents and teachers are trained in evidence-based practices for inclusive education and autism support. Parents and teachers then work together in cooperative groups to implement learned practices and also implement these practices at home and in their classrooms. Programming for Syrian refugee families in Turkey includes teacher trainings in inclusive education. Parent trainings aim to foster healthy home environments for affected children. In addition, sessions are designed to facilitate family and teacher support, self-development groups, and community education to increase understanding of trauma and autism. The programmatic components are standardized but are tailored to the composition of the group and the target setting, be it in the classroom, home, or community.

4.1. Parent & Teacher Training Cooperatives

Parents and teachers of primary-school-aged children are trained in globally recognized evidence-based practices for supporting their children with autism at home and in the community. Particular emphasis is placed on developing and improving independent methods of communication, reducing challenging behaviors, and teaching new skills.

4.2. Parent, Teacher, and Sibling Support and Self-Development Groups

These groups provide participants with safe spaces to share and reflect upon their experiences of supporting trauma-affected loved ones and loved ones with autism while gaining a deeper understanding of the experiences of those affected. Participants increase their self-confidence, improve their self-care, and discover ways to integrate their strengths and interests into their daily lives.

4.3. Community Education

These sessions educate community members about autism and trauma in order to reduce community stigma and increase understanding. They are offered to doctors, teachers, government officials, and general community members in order to decrease the marginalization of these individuals within these communities.

5. Impact of Gendered Challenges on Interventions

The instabilities inherent in refugee life pose a number of challenges for the organization's effective implementation of programming. The gender challenges identified significantly impact A Global Voice for Autism's ability to carry out educational interventions for trauma-affected children in the following ways:

5.1. Attendance and Participation

Attrition rates for participating families and teachers in A Global Voice for Autism's programs in Turkey are high. The most frequently reported reasons for attrition are "required by spouse" and "inability to access program." In the attrition cases in the past Turkey programs, 78% occurred in families where a family member had reported issues of domestic violence. Incidents at home, which often interlink challenges to masculinity with domestic and/or sexual violence, are primary reasons for attrition and, therefore, inhibitors to the success of the program [38]. Furthermore, these experiences and challenges pre-occupy families and take precedence over program participation. In order to attend and actively participate in the program, families must have their primary needs met [39].

5.2. Counterproductive Modeling and Behavioral Strategies

Modeling is a common behavior for children. When children see unhealthy and violent coping mechanisms at home, they may practice these behaviors. This is a particular issue when it comes to the interventions that are used, many of which rely on teaching through modeling skills and reinforcement of modeling behavior. Furthermore, consistency is key to the efficacy of these strategies, and when violence or parental disengagement occurs at home, it limits the efficacy of the home-based interventions in support of the education of trauma-affected children [40].

5.3. Trauma Replication

Existing trauma for trauma-affected children is perpetuated and exacerbated by instability in the home. As one of the strongest predictors of child performance, adverse childhood experiences (ACEs), such as domestic violence, parental disengagement, and displacement affect a child's ability to learn new skills and engage with their environments [40,41]. Outcomes of these ACEs can include lack of trust. In order for educational interventions for trauma-affected children to be effective, trust of parent and teacher caregivers is essential [42].

6. Recommendations

Based on the aforementioned gendered challenges to educational interventions in the Syrian refugee population in Turkey, the following are recommended:

1. Refugee support organizations should advocate for a policy within Turkey that provides refugees seeking emergency support services, such as psychological support, legal support, and domestic and sexual violence support, with status immunity. This means that no refugee or "guest" will risk deportation or punitive measures when accessing these support services.
2. In concurrence with the above policy recommendation, there should be the establishment of a network of existing organizations that agree to support all refugees in need, regardless of their legal status, so that parents and teachers can access the services they need in order to achieve a level of wellbeing that enables them to effectively support children with autism and trauma-affected children.
3. A Global Voice for Autism, and other organizations supporting educational interventions in Syrian refugee populations in Turkey, should increasingly integrate their support for affected children with parental support programs that teach parents to address their own trauma so that they can focus on addressing the needs of their children. Such programs will be self-reinforcing

because, as parents reach a level where they are able to implement effective practices in support of their children, parenting will become easier and parenting stress will decrease.
4. In order to address the isolation experienced by many refugee mothers, as well as the lack of safe spaces for fathers to discuss trauma, partnerships should be established with other community organizations to expand the availability of women's and men's groups for parents of trauma-affected children to create spaces for connection and experience processing with others who have similar experiences.

7. Conclusions

The creation of stable, secure environments for children is essential to the success of educational interventions for trauma-affected refugee children. Trauma alters the brain in ways that result in learning differences, and a sense of security is integral to effective trauma-informed education and care. In the Syrian refugee population in Turkey, creating these secure environments for learning is a challenge due to gender-related issues of masculinity, domestic violence, and sexual violence. This, in conjunction with the persistent structural issues in existing support systems, inhibit access to appropriate support for the population. In order to address these issues, and to foster safe environments where stakeholders can support trauma-affected children in their education, policies in Turkey must ensure the safety of refugees who access support services. Organizations must also maintain refugee confidentiality regardless of legal status, and A Global Voice for Autism and other community organizations must increasingly integrate parent trauma support into child trauma support trainings while providing access to networks of support for both men and women caregivers in the community.

To achieve such results, the availability of funding and resources must be discussed. In 2016, the European Union (EU) signed an agreement with Turkey to assume responsibility for migrants who initially entered Europe through Turkey. It was intended to limit the influx of families entering the EU through Turkey. The EU allocated three billion Euros in aid to Turkey to assist Syrian migrant communities. However, there is concern that the majority of funds have been allocated to the administrative costs of international civil society organizations rather than to direct aid for the refugees [43]. A comprehensive review should be undertaken to ascertain how the funding has been allocated to date, with the development of a strategy to promote program collaboration outlined above to enhance the direct care of Syrian refugee children.

Finally, though the difficulties faced by refugee children are immense, there is a growing international awareness that action needs to be taken to address displacement related challenges. In 2016, the UN General Assembly adopted the New York Declaration for Refugees and Migrants [44]. In 2018, the Global Compact for Safe, Orderly and Regular Migration and the Compact on Refugees were finalized [45]. Together they hopefully provide a global framework to support international efforts to address the crisis. It will be imperative that the United Nations focuses on the efforts in Turkey so as to operationalize the Compacts and optimize the care of Syrian children in Turkey.

Author Contributions: M.D. contributions include the conceptualization, methodology, investigation, formal analysis, writing—original draft material, reviewing and editing, and project administration. C.O. contributions include conceptualization, analysis, writing—original article, and reviewing and editing.

Funding: This research received no external funding.

Acknowledgments: The authors would like to acknowledge the Syrian families and children who struggle with the aftermath of conflict, war, violence, displacement, and trauma.

Conflicts of Interest: The authors declare no conflict of interest.

References

1. Boyden, J.; de Berry, J. Children in Adversity. *Forced Migr. Rev.* **2000**, *9*, 33–36.
2. Syria's Mental Health Crisis. Brookings Institute. 2016. Available online: https://www.brookings.edu/blog/future-development/2016/04/25/syrias-mental-health-crisis/ (accessed on 15 August 2019).

3. A Global Voice for Autism. 2017. 27 September 2019. Available online: http://www.aglobalvoiceforautism.org.
4. Saakvitne, K.W.; Gamble, S.; Pearlman, L.A.; Lev, B.T. *Risking Connection: A Training Curriculum for Working with Survivors of Childhood Abuse*; The Sidran Press: Baltimore, MD, USA, 2000.
5. Lyon, D.M.; Parker, K.J.; Katz, M.; Schartzberg, A.F. Developmental cascades linking stress inoculation, regulation and resilience. *Front. Behav. Neurosci.* **2009**, *3*, 32. [CrossRef] [PubMed]
6. Johnson, E.O.; Kamilaris, T.C.; Chrousos, G.P.; Gold, P.W. Mechanisms of stress: A dynamic overview of hormonal and behavioral homeostasis. *Rev. Neurosci. Biobehav. Rev.* **1992**, *16*, 115–130. [CrossRef]
7. Fortin, A. The meaning of protection in the refugee definition. *Int. J. Refug. Law* **2000**, *14*, 548–576. [CrossRef]
8. George, J. Migration traumatic experiences and refugee distress-implications for social work practices. *Clin. Soc. Work. J.* **2012**, *40*, 429–437. [CrossRef]
9. El-Khani, A.; Ulph, F.; Peters, S.; Calam, R. Syria-the challenges of parenting in refugee situations of immediate displacement. *Intervention* **2016**, *14*, 99–113. [CrossRef]
10. Women's Refugee Commission; International Refugee Committee. *Disabilities Among Refugees and Conflict-Affected Populations*; Women's Refugee Commission: New York, NY, USA; International Refugee Committee: New York, NY, USA, 2008.
11. Imanaka, A.; Morinobu, S.; Toki, S.; Yamawaki, S. Importance of early environment in the development of post-traumatic stress disorder-like behaviors. *Behav. Brain Res.* **2006**, *173*, 129–137. [CrossRef]
12. Shonkoff, J.P.; Garner, A.S.; Committee on Psychosocial Aspects of Child and Family Health; Committee on Early Childhood, Adoption and Dependent Care; Section on Developmental and Behavioral Pediatrics; Siegel, B.S.; Wood, D.L. The Lifelong Effects of Early Childhood Adversity and Toxic Stress. *Pediatrics* **2012**, *129*, e232–e246. [CrossRef]
13. UN Security Council. Conflict-Related Sexual Violence-Report of the Secretary General. 2015. Available online: http://reliefweb.int/report/world/conflict-related-sexual-violence-report-secretary-general-s2015203-enar (accessed on 14 August 2019).
14. Ending Rape as A Weapon of War: A Multi—Country Initiative, MADRE. Available online: https://www.madre.org/initiatives/ending-rape-weapon-war (accessed on 15 August 2019).
15. Tackling Honor Killings through Sexual and Gender Rights Advocacy-Recommendations for Policy and Practice, Centre for Transnational Development and Collaboration (CTDC). Available online: http://ctdc.org/publication/tackling-honour-killings-sexual-gender-rights-advocacy-recommendations-policy-practice/ (accessed on 15 August 2019).
16. Sev'er, A.; Yurdakul, G. Culture of honor, culture of change-a feminist analysis of honor killings in rural Turkey. *Violence Women* **2001**, *7*, 964–998. [CrossRef]
17. Storr, W. The Rape of Men: The Darkest Secret of War. *The Guardian*, 2011. Available online: https://www.theguardian.com/society/2011/jul/17/the-rape-of-men (accessed on 14 August 2019).
18. Hynes, M.; Cardozo, B.P. Observations from the CDC-Sexual violence against refugee women. *J. Women's Health Gend.-Based Med.* **2004**, *9*, 891. [CrossRef]
19. Save the Children. *Futures under Threat-the Impact of the Educational Crisis on Syria's Children*; Save the Children: London, UK, 2014.
20. New York Times. Domestic Violence on the Rise among Syrian Refugees. 2014. Available online: https://kristof.blogs.nytimes.com/2014/08/29/domestic-violence-on-the-rise-among-syrian-refugees/?_r=0 (accessed on 27 September 2019).
21. *The Cost of War: Calculating the Impact of the Collapse of Syria's Education System on Syria's Future*; American Institute for Research: Washington, DC, USA, Save The Children: London, UK, 2015; Available online: https://resourcecentre.savethechildren.net/library/cost-war-calculating-impact-collapse-syrias-education-system-syrias-future (accessed on 14 August 2019).
22. Letsch, C. Women's rights and gender equity, Syria's Refugees-Fears of Abuse Grow as Turkish Men Snap up Wives. *The Guardian*, 2014. Available online: https://www.theguardian.com/world/2014/sep/08/syrian-refugee-brides-turkish-husbands-marriage (accessed on 5 September 2015).
23. Diamond, M.; Robinson, K.; Statham, S. Issue Brief-Turkey Programs De-Identified Family Data. *The Global Voice for Autism*, 2017.
24. Koss, M. Blame, shame and community-justice responses to violence against women. *Am. Psychol.* **2000**, *55*, 1332–1343. [CrossRef] [PubMed]

25. El-Bushra, J.; Smith, E.R. *Gender, Education and Peacebuilding-A Review of Selected Learning for Peace Case Studies*; UNICEF: New York, NY, USA, June 2016.
26. UNESCO. *Migration, Displacement and Education: Building Bridges, Not Walls. Global Education Monitoring Report Summary*; UNESCO: Paris, France, 2019.
27. Five Unique Challenges Facing Syrian Refugee Women. Concern Worldwide, U.S. 2016. Available online: http://www.concernusa.org/story/five-unique-challenges-facing-syrian-refugee-women/ (accessed on 15 August 2019).
28. Mackenzie, C.; McDowell, C.; Pittaway, E. Beyond "Do no Harm". *J. Refug. Stud.* **2007**, *20*, 299–319. [CrossRef]
29. Farris, E.M.; Mohamed, H.S. Picturing immigration-how the media criminalizes immigrants. *Politics Groups Identities* **2018**, *6*, 814–824. [CrossRef]
30. Carroll, C. The European Refugee Crisis and the Myth of the Immigrant Rapist. *EuropeNow Research*, 2017. Available online: https://www.europenowjournal.org/2017/07/05/untitled/ (accessed on 5 September 2015).
31. Keedi, A.; Yaghi, Z.; Barker, G. *We Can. Never Go Back to How Things Were Before-A Qualitative Study on War, Masculinities, and Gender Relations with Lebanese and Syrian Refugee Men and Women*; ABAAD: Beirut, Lebanon; Promundo: Washington, DC, USA, May 2017.
32. Wong, C.; Odom, S.; Hume, K.; Cox, A.W.; Fettig, A.; Kucharczyk, S.; Brock, M.E.; Plavnick, J.B.; Fleury, V.P.; Schultz, T.R. Evidence-based practices for children, youth, and young adults with autism spectrum disorder: A comprehensive review. *J. Autism Dev. Discord* **2015**, *45*, 1951–1966. [CrossRef] [PubMed]
33. *Gender Analysis in of Syrian Refugee Parents*; Unpublished Data; A Global Voice for Autism: Minneapolis, MN, USA, 2017.
34. Oberg, C.N. Embracing International Children's Rights—From Policy to Practice. *Clin. Pediatr.* **2012**, *51*, 619–624. [CrossRef]
35. Hjern, A.; Bouvier, P. Migrant children-a challenge for European paediatricians. *Acta Paediatr.* **2007**, *93*, 1535–1539. [CrossRef]
36. Disaster and Emergency Management Authority (AFAD). Syrian Women in Turkey. 2014. Available online: https://www.afad.gov.tr/upload/Node/3904/xfiles/afad-suriye-kdn_eng.pdf (accessed on 15 August 2015).
37. IRIN. US Probe into Turkey-Syria Aid Corruption Deepens. 2016. Available online: https://www.irinnews.org/investigations/2016/05/09/us-probe-turkey-syria-aid-corruption-deepens (accessed on 27 September 2019).
38. Diamond, M.; Robinson, K.; Statham, S. Turkey Programs De-Identified Family Data. Unpublished.
39. Population in Movement: Addressing the Opportunities and Challenges to Ensure Care and Services to the Migrants with Autism and Developmental Disabilities, United Nations. 2017. Available online: http://webtv.un.org/watch/population-in-movement-addressing-the-opportunities-and-challenges-to-ensure-care-and-services-to-the-migrants-with-autism-and-developmental-disabilities/5380885058001 (accessed on 15 August 2015).
40. Centers for Disease Control and Prevention. Centers for Disease Control and Prevention. Adverse Childhood Experiences; Centers for Disease Control and Prevention: Atlanta, GA, USA. In *Adverse Childhood Experiences*; Centers for Disease Control and Prevention: Atlanta, GA, USA, 2019. Available online: https://www.cdc.gov/violenceprevention/childabuseandneglect/acestudy/index.html (accessed on 15 August 2015).
41. Hunt, T.K.A.; Slack, K.S.; Berger, L.M. Adverse childhood experiences and behavioral problems in middle childhood. *Child. Abus. Negl.* **2017**, *67*, 391–402. [CrossRef]
42. Menschner, C.; Maul, A. *Issue Brief-Key Ingredients for Successful Trauma-Informed Care Implementation*; Center for Health Care Strategies, Inc., The Robert Wood Johnson Foundation: Trenton, NJ, USA, April 2016.
43. Sirkeci, I. Turkey's refugees, Syrian and refugees from Turkey-a country of insecurity. *Migr. Lett.* **2017**, *1*, 127–144. [CrossRef]
44. Seifman, R. Refugees, migrant, and displaced populations: The United Nations New York Declaration and the WHO International Health Regulations. *Int. Health* **2017**, *9*, 325–326. [CrossRef]
45. Turk, V.; Garlick, M. From burden and responsibilities to opportunities-the compressive refugee framework ad a global compact on refugees. *Int. J. Refug. Law* **2016**, *28*, 656–678. [CrossRef]

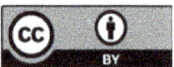

© 2019 by the authors. Licensee MDPI, Basel, Switzerland. This article is an open access article distributed under the terms and conditions of the Creative Commons Attribution (CC BY) license (http://creativecommons.org/licenses/by/4.0/).

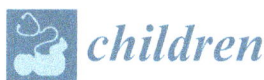

Opinion

Challenges in Caring for Linguistic Minorities in the Pediatric Population

Logan DeBord [1,*], Kali Ann Hopkins [2] and Padma Swamy [3]

1. Department of Dermatology, School of Medicine, University of Colorado, Anschutz Cancer Pavilion Building, 3rd Floor, 1665 Aurora Court, Aurora, CO 80045, USA
2. Department of Pediatrics, Feinberg School of Medicine, Northwestern University, 225 E Chicago Ave, Chicago, IL 60611, USA
3. Department of Pediatrics, Baylor College of Medicine, 8080 N. Stadium Drive, Houston, TX 77054, USA
* Correspondence: logan.debord@utexas.edu

Received: 10 June 2019; Accepted: 22 July 2019; Published: 25 July 2019

Abstract: Physicians in the United States (U.S.) face unique obstacles in providing care for persons with limited English proficiency (LEP), especially speakers of rare languages. Lack of professional resources is not a problem exclusive to health care delivery, with speakers of Mayan dialects receiving increasingly narrow representation in detention centers and immigration courts at the U.S.–Mexico border. Parent-child dynamics and other crucial information related to pediatric care may be lost in translation in the event of inadequate interpreter services. Several strategies could address disparities in medical care faced by persons with LEP, speaking rare as well as more common languages. These include increasing the availability of professional interpreters via expanded and/or incentivized training programs, providing focused education in interpreter services for medical students, and unifying interpretation services provided by local consulates and nonprofit agencies for both medical and legal purposes.

Keywords: limited English proficiency (LEP); linguistic minorities; medical interpreters; immigrants; refugees; Mayan

1. Introduction

The current United States (U.S.) population was built on the foundations of a rich immigration history. While English remains the unofficial language in practice, approximately 21.6% of U.S. residents ages 5 and older speak another language primarily at home, according to the U.S. Census [1]. An executive order released in 2000 mandated that federal agencies improve systems and programs for Limited English Proficiency (LEP) individuals; in 2003, the Department of Health and Human Services (HHS) published guidelines on how to address the order [2,3]. The HHS required that health care entities take "reasonable steps to provide meaningful access to each individual with limited English proficiency eligible to be served or likely to be encountered in its health programs and activities" [4]. According to Jacobs et al., there are no federal guidelines requiring certified or licensed interpreters. While not mandated, HHS does encourage the use of certified medical interpreters [2]. In the U.S., there are two accreditation bodies that provide certification for medical interpreters: the National Board of Certification for Medical Interpreters and the Certification Commission for Healthcare Interpreters [2]. However, interpretation is costly and sometimes difficult to implement in small clinics which essentially function as businesses [4]. However, several state-run versions of our federal insurance program will reimburse health care/language services for use of interpreters [4].

While this provision broadly refers to all interpretation, we encountered two situations in which the existing system to connect patients with trained interpreters failed. While pantomiming or using ad hoc interpreters may be tempting in the setting of a busy teaching environment, one meta-analysis showed that quality of care for limited English proficient patients is inferior with the use of such untrained interpreters [5]. Lack of proficiency in a patient's native language commonly results in errors of medical interpretation, with potential clinical consequences [6]. Even Spanish-speaking patients in the United States have been found to suffer reduced clinical encounter time and substandard treatment compared to native English speakers [7]. However, language services are legally mandated to be available free-of-charge to patients in facilities that receive federal funding. The first situation that we encountered (described by L.D.) details a challenge in caring for a speaker of a rare language despite having a fairly robust interpretation service program in place. The second situation (described by K.A.H.) gives insight into a common practice by providers when faced with language difficulties and was encountered in a resource-limited setting outside the U.S.

2. A Shortage of Qualified Interpreters in Rare Languages (L.D.)

I was a third-year medical student conducting vaccinations at a children's mobile clinic that delivers care to patients who are often under- or uninsured. Most of these patients were recipients of Medicaid, which is our combined federal and state government insurance program that addresses medical costs for those with low income. Many patients in our mobile clinic were also recent immigrants to the U.S. with limited English proficiency. Such was the case when a newly arrived Guatemalan child presented to the clinic with his father, who spoke their primary language of an uncommon Mayan dialect in addition to very rudimentary Spanish. This problem compounded unravelling the child's chief complaint of headache for our health care team.

Having rotated extensively in our county hospital, I was confident in my ability to have a Spanish translator, either in person or via phone, at a patient's bedside within minutes. However, medical interpreters in rare languages are more difficult to find. Often a scheduled appointment is required weeks in advance. Our team resorted to relying on the father's broken Spanish, which was then translated into English via an on-demand Spanish phone interpreter. However, I noted some discomfort in the boy's responses to our probing questions: had he seen anything disturbing during the journey? Was he satisfied with the meals that his father was able to provide?

Additionally, it also became apparent that not all of our questions were being understood by the father once translated from English to Spanish. My attending physician (P.S.) decided that on this visit, our priority should be to screen for *red flag* symptoms of headache that might signal intracranial pathology. We were sufficiently comfortable in our determination via interview that the headaches were not occipital in location, did not awaken the child from sleep, and were not accompanied by nausea, vomiting, or ataxia. We also completed a neurological exam, which revealed the absence of focal weakness, papilledema and nuchal rigidity. My attending physician ultimately decided to schedule an interpreter in their native language and reassess the situation at a follow-up visit in two weeks. I left clinic that day wondering about the factors contributing to the child's suffering. Would fluency in his native tongue have allowed us to pick up on nuances that might be key to the diagnosis?

This recent interaction with the father and his son resulted in my becoming aware of the obstacles in providing care for persons with limited English proficiency in my home country. Lack of professional resources for persons with LEP is not a problem exclusive to health care delivery, with speakers of Mayan dialects also receiving increasingly narrow representation in detention centers and immigration courts at our Southern border [8].

3. Risks of Playing the Telephone Game with Medical Information (K.A.H.)

As an Internal Medicine-Pediatrics resident rotating at a teaching hospital in Kenya, I arrived in a setting in which trained interpreters do not exist. My team was rounding in the "failure-to-thrive room," which was slightly bigger than a closet and crowded with five patients and their mothers. During rounds, we diagnosed a child with visceral leishmaniasis, but his mother spoke only a rare tribal language. Fortunately, another mother in the room also spoke this language, and we found a nursing student who spoke this second mother's primary tribal language, in addition to Swahili.

In the end, the team translated my English to Swahili, and then to both tribal languages. Aware of the potential pitfalls of *playing telephone* with medical information, I shortened the message to the diagnosis, its method of transmission, the prognosis, and treatment. The mother eventually nodded in understanding that her son would likely recover, as long as he could receive antibiotics in the hospital for an additional three weeks.

4. Options to Address Shortcomings in Care for U.S. Residents with Limited English Proficiency

While not ideal, interactions such as these may avoid the consequence of minimal understanding for patients in a resource-limited setting. However, inherent structural and attitudinal barriers underlie a lack of access to qualified interpreters for both Spanish speakers and speakers of rare languages alike in the United States. Our country currently lacks a required standardized training and certification process for medical interpreters, which increases the likelihood of preventable medical errors in the care of such patients [9]. The rigors of medical training leave little time for trainees to become proficient in another language, despite many being surrounded by non-English speakers during clinical rotations. In medical schools, there is widespread instruction on the need to always use a qualified interpreter but seldom advanced discussions regarding how to advocate for linguistic minorities. As we have learned, essential parent-child dynamics, as well as patient-provider rapport, may also be lost in translation when playing games of *medical telephone*.

Several possible solutions can address disparities in care faced by both patients and parents with LEP. Increasing the number and availability of professional interpreters is paramount to minimizing clinical consequences for such minorities. One study supports the notion that requiring at least 100 training hours for interpreters would likely significantly reduce errors in medical interpretation [10]. From our personal experience, we observed that patients generally seemed more satisfied when speaking to an interpreter visible via videoconference compared to telephone, a finding which was reflected in a previous study [9]. In terms of medical students' competency in using available interpreter services, focused education likely results in earlier proficiency compared to those who receive no training [11]. Incorporating translator difficulties, particularly in pediatric encounters in which there is both the perspective of the patient and guardian to consider, into patient simulations in medical training might be beneficial to prepare for real-life scenarios.

For rare languages in particular, outsourcing hospital-based medical interpretation to call centers in foreign countries may be a key strategy to provide access independent of the patient's location [12]. However, a more pragmatic method might be to address problems in our health care and legal systems simultaneously. Increasing Mayan-language interpreter courses could bolster the number of qualified interpreters at a time when demand is expected to increase in both immigration courts, safety net clinics, and other community settings [13,14]. Unifying interpretation services provided by local consulates and nonprofit agencies for both medical and legal purposes could ensure that speakers of uncommon Central American dialects receive adequate representation.

Pediatricians in training should be aware that difficulties in interpretation can add to the challenge of untangling already-complex relationships between the patient and guardian. In our patient encounter at the mobile clinic, we were aware of the possibility that the boy might not be willing to admit that he was hungry or thirsty in front of his father. Ready accessibility of an interpreter in the patient's primary language is even more important in these types of scenarios. When this is not possible, efforts should be made to rule out life-threatening etiologies of the chief complaint while scheduling adequate follow-up with a qualified interpreter.

Educating medical students to the breadth of challenges faced by linguistic minorities via clinical exposure, didactics by certified interpreters, and patient simulations would prepare them to advocate for these patients in their future careers. Simultaneously, local and federal agencies should mandate a standardized certification process for interpreters and implement incentives for entry into the field. This dual approach would ensure that pediatric patients have their voices heard in an increasingly global environment.

Acknowledgments: We acknowledge editing support from the Baylor College of Medicine Compliance & Audit Services for the purpose of maintaining patient privacy and confidentiality.

Conflicts of Interest: The authors declare no conflict of interest.

References

1. Ingraham, C. Millions of U.S. citizens don't speak English to one another. That's not a problem. *The Washington Post (Economic Policy)* **2018**. Available online: https://www.washingtonpost.com/news/wonk/wp/2018/05/21/millions-of-u-s-citizens-dont-speak-english-to-each-other-thats-not-a-problem/?noredirect=on&utm_term=.a9ce96263ff3 (accessed on 21 July 2019).
2. Jacobs, B.; Ryan, A.M.; Henrichs, K.S.; Weiss, B.D. Medical interpreters in outpatient practice. *Ann. Fam. Med.* **2018**, *16*, 70–76. [CrossRef] [PubMed]
3. Department of Health and Human Services. Guidance to federal financial assistance recipients regarding Title VI prohibition against national origin discrimination affecting limited English proficient persons. *Fed. Regist.* **2003**, *68*, 47311. Available online: https://www.govinfo.gov/content/pkg/FR-2003-08-08/pdf/03-20179.pdf (accessed on 21 July 2019).
4. Department of Health and Human Services. Nondiscrimination in Health Programs and Activities. *Fed. Regist.* **2016**, *92*, 31375–31473. Available online: https://www.federalregister.gov/documents/2016/05/18/2016-11458/nondiscrimination-in-health-programs-and-activities (accessed on 21 July 2019).
5. Flores, G. The impact of medical interpreter services on the quality of health care: a systematic review. *Med. Care Res. Rev.* **2005**, *62*, 255–299. [CrossRef] [PubMed]
6. Flores, G.; Laws, M.B.; Mayo, S.J.; Zuckerman, B.; Abreu, M.; Medina, L.; Hardt, E.J. Errors in medical interpretation and their potential clinical consequences in pediatric encounters. *Pediatrics* **2003**, *111*, 6–14. [CrossRef] [PubMed]
7. VanderWielen, L.M.; Enurah, A.S.; Rho, H.Y.; Nagarkatti-Gude, D.R.; Michelsen-King, P.; Crossman, S.H.; Vanderbilt, A.A. Medical interpreters: Improvements to address access, equity, and quality of care for limited-English-proficient patients. *Acad. Med.* **2014**, *89*, 1324–1327. [CrossRef] [PubMed]
8. Connolly, C. Mayan language survives in Champaign, poses challenge in immigration court. *Chicago Tribune (News)* **2017**. Available online: http://www.chicagotribune.com/news/immigration/ct-met-immigrants-mayan-languages-20170926-story.html (accessed on 21 July 2019).
9. Schulz, T.R.; Leder, K.; Akinci, I.; Biggs, B.-A. Improvements in patient care: Videoconferencing to improve access to interpreters during clinical consultations for refugee and immigrant patients. *Aust. Health Rev.* **2015**, *39*, 395–399. [CrossRef] [PubMed]
10. Flores, G.; Abreu, M.; Barone, C.P.; Bachur, R.; Lin, H. Errors of medical interpretation and their potential clinical consequences: a comparison of professional versus ad hoc versus no interpreters. *Ann. Emerg. Med.* **2012**, *60*, 545–553. [CrossRef] [PubMed]
11. Omoruyi, E.A.; Dunkle, J.; Dendy, C.; McHugh, E.; Barratt, M.S. Cross Talk: Evaluation of a curriculum to teach medical students how to use telephone interpreter services. *Acad. Pediatr.* **2018**, *18*, 214–219. [CrossRef] [PubMed]
12. Silverman, L. When patients speak French, Hindi Or Nepali, medical interpreters step in. *KERA News* **2017**. Available online: http://keranews.org/post/when-patients-speak-french-hindi-or-nepali-medical-interpreters-step (accessed on 21 July 2019).
13. Carcamo, C. Ancient Mayan languages are creating problems for today's immigration courts. *Los Angeles Times* **2016**. Available online: http://www.latimes.com/local/california/la-me-mayan-indigenous-languages-20160725-snap-story.html (accessed on 21 July 2019).
14. Lo Wang, H. Language barriers pose challenges for Mayan migrant children. *National Public Radio (All Things Considered)* **2014**. Available online: https://www.npr.org/sections/codeswitch/2014/07/01/326426927/language-barriers-pose-challenges-for-mayan-migrant-children (accessed on 21 July 2019).

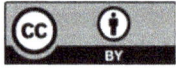

© 2019 by the authors. Licensee MDPI, Basel, Switzerland. This article is an open access article distributed under the terms and conditions of the Creative Commons Attribution (CC BY) license (http://creativecommons.org/licenses/by/4.0/).

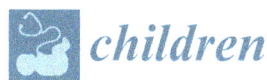

Case Report

The Use of Age Assessment in the Context of Child Migration: Imprecise, Inaccurate, Inconclusive and Endangers Children's Rights

Ranit Mishori

Department of Family Medicine, Georgetown University School of Medicine, Washington, DC 20007, USA; mishorir@georgetown.edu

Received: 1 July 2019; Accepted: 22 July 2019; Published: 23 July 2019

Abstract: Anecdotal reports suggest migrant children at the US border have had to undergo age assessment procedures to prove to immigration officials they qualify for special protections afforded to those under age 18. There are a variety of methods to assess the chronological ages of minors, including imaging studies such as X-rays of the wrist, teeth, or collarbone. However, these procedures have come under great scrutiny for being arbitrary and inaccurate, with a significant margin of error, because they are generally based on reference materials that do not take into account ethnicity, nutritional status, disease, and developmental history, considerations which are especially relevant for individuals coming from conflict and/or resource-constrained environments. Using these procedures for migration purposes represent an unethical use of science and medicine, which can potentially deprive minors with the protections that they are owed under US and international laws, and which may have devastating consequences. We should advocate for the creation special protocols, educate law enforcement and legal actors, ensure such procedures are carried out only as a last resort and by independent actors, emphasize child protection and always put the child's best interest at the core.

Keywords: age assessments; migration; child-protection; medico-legal ethics; forensic evaluations

---

1. Introduction

A 17-year-old teenage boy fleeing gang violence in Honduras was apprehended by the U.S. Border Patrol in Texas and placed in detention in Arizona. Though he informed detention staff of his age, they accused him of lying and placed him in an adult facility, where adult detainees threatened and harassed him over his $5.00 telephone card. He once again told the authorities that he did not belong in the adult facility. They said: Prove it. Detention staff took him to the prison clinic for a dental exam, which was interpreted to indicate that he was 16–17 years old, so he was subsequently transferred to an age-appropriate facility. He was evaluated by a clinical psychologist who conducted a forensic evaluation for his asylum case, documenting psychiatric symptoms and psychological effects of the gang violence he had experienced. His asylum case is still pending.

This story seems like a positive example of science and medicine in service of child protection. However, the dental assessment, with its two-year margin of error range, could easily have gone the other way, and caused an adolescent to be inappropriately placed in an adult facility, without the procedural and substantive protections due to minors under U.S. and international law.

2. What Are Age Assessments?

Age assessments generally refer to any procedures used to establish an individual's chronological age—the age from the day that person was born. Chronological age is, in and of itself, of limited value in predicting maturity, social or intellectual ability, or a person's capacity to function in a new environment.

There are a variety of methods to assess the chronological ages of minors [1]. From history taking, to a medical examination (physical exam, sexual maturity); the use of official state documents; Anthropometric evaluation (measurements of height, weight, head circumference); imaging studies—X-rays of the wrist, teeth, or collarbone, or MRIs [2]. Table 1 offers a review of these methods and associated information.

Table 1. Different methods for age assessments.

Non Medical	How It Is Done; by Whom	Possible Issues
Documentation	Retrieve, review, and request documents such as a birth certificate, immunization record, or others that might have the child's DOB.	• Many children will not have any papers; papers get lost. • There are no standards on documentation of identity or age. • Contacting family members in the home country may be an option in trying to retrieve official state documents.
Interview and history taking	Use the history and patient/client narrative, or any family member to try to assess the year of birth of the child in question.	• Avoid an intimidating style of interview. • Allow only professionals with training to elicit this information. • There are no specific protocols on how to conduct such interviews.
Medical No one should rely on physical appearance to determine a child's chronological age, as there are significant variations in physical development.		
Physical—sexual maturity	Use standard protocols for sexual maturity assessment such as Taner Staging [3].	• Taner staging may be less useful in late adolescence and in those with an early onset of puberty. • Visual inspections can be traumatic to children, especially those who may have experienced sexual violence. • Never take pictures without adhering to thorough consent processes.
Physical—anthropomorphic	Use height, weight, skin rating, and compare to reference values [4,5].	Such measurements often do not reflect variations due to race, ethnicity, nutritional status, and socio-economic status.
Imaging Studies They rely on skeletal changes that occur as children's bones mature; significant bias exists in interpretation and such imaging studies can never report the precise chronological age of a child. Variations range is generally accepted to be +2/−2 years [6].		
Radiological Tests—(carpal) hand and wrist X-rays	Assess the fusing progression of carpal bones.	• The most common method used. • Data relies on populations samples that do not reflect diversity of race, ethnicity, nutritional status, and SE background. • There are no standards for specific populations (Latino, African, and Middle Eastern). • Radiation exposure.
Radiology Dental X-rays	Relies on presence, absence, or development of the roots of the 3rd molars.	• Data relies on populations samples that do not reflect diversity of race, ethnicity, nutritional status, and SE background. • There are no standards for specific populations. • Radiation exposure.
Radiology: Collar bone X-rays	Assesses the fusing process of the clavicle.	• Data relies on populations samples that do not reflect diversity of race, ethnicity, nutritional status, and SE background. • There are no standards for specific populations. • Radiation exposure.
MRI of the knee or hand [7,8]	It has been suggested as a method to counter the ethical problems with X-ray use and avoid radiation [8].	• Attracting increasing attention. • Concerns for incidental findings and follow up. • More expensive.

(Adapted from the Position Paper on Age Assessment in the Context of Separated Children in Europe 2012) [9].

As a clinical procedure, skeletal age assessments are used frequently in pediatric endocrinology [10]. Dental age assessments have been used, among other things, for international adoptions [11]. These radiographs of the dental crown and root of the third molar tooth are compared with reference studies to determine age. Similarly, hand and wrist radiographs are compared to radiographs from reference studies in order to judge skeletal age and bone maturation. However, multiple studies have concluded that both methods are only able to produce estimates within a range of at least two years. Research studies have demonstrated that these methods systematically under and over estimate ages [12–14].

Imaging tests have come under great scrutiny for being arbitrary and inaccurate, with a significant margin of error [12,13]. This is mostly because they are generally based on reference materials that do not take into account ethnicity, nutritional status, disease, and developmental history, considerations that are especially relevant for individuals coming from conflict and/or resource-constrained environments. Other concerns are that these tests are invasive, expensive, and potentially harmful exposing minors to unnecessary radiation.

These inaccurate procedures represent an unethical and unprofessional use of science and medicine for procedures that are both inconclusive and can potentially deprive those under the age of 18 with the protections that they are owed under the US and international human rights laws. Inaccurate assessments may have devastating consequences for children who may suddenly be 'determined' to be an adult, thus denied special protection and other human rights provisions. Such protections usually include protection from abuse, abandonment, and neglect and codified requirements to promote children's safety, education, health, and nutrition, and protect them from exploitation and abuse [15,16].

For example, being moved to an adult detention center without appropriate services for minors and where their safety may be at risk is counter to child-protection provisions. Other examples under US law include loss of the right to non-adversarial asylum proceedings, limits on duration of detention, and support for reunification with parents and other relatives [15,16].

3. What Can We Do?

There are no standardized protocols in the US meant to offer guidance regarding the use of age assessment methods for minors. It is imperative that they be developed with input from physicians, social workers, human rights experts, and other stakeholders who can review possible scenarios through a child-protection lens.

As clinicians and as human rights defenders, we must first acknowledge, and ensure others are aware, that the determination of the chronological age of a child is almost never accurate or precise. It is not an exact science. In the context of migration (as opposed to pediatric endocrinology, for example) there are significant social consequences and potential risk to the safety of the minor whose age is being assessed or disputed. While in some medical contexts there is merit to such testing, in legal contexts it is a more dubious practice. Therefore, age assessments for migration purposes, especially via radiologic imaging, should be carried out only as a last resort.

Key considerations must be given to who should have a mandate to request these tests, and for what reasons. Motivation and reasoning may vary based on the requesting entity: Border patrol, governmental agents, representatives of the judicial system handing asylum cases, social workers, and physicians. Not all of these stakeholders may have the child's best interest at heart, or the intention and means of ensuring child protection above all.

If or when age assessment procedures are ordered, they must be carried out by independent professionals and those who have expertise in performing them and interpreting them appropriately; by professionals who are familiar with genetic, medical, and ethnic variations, and differences in cultural background. We should strive to create protocols that specify (or even restrict) who is allowed to refer minors for or order age assessments.

When considering whether to subject a child to an age assessment, evaluators should balance physical, developmental, psychological, cultural, and environmental factors. They must never force such assessments on minors, must avoid invasive or intrusive exams and must always choose the least invasive assessment first.

Consent protocols should be followed, and informed consent must be obtained every time for these procedures in accordance with common pediatric guidelines [17]. Protections must be developed to ensure that minors are never forced, coerced, or pressured to undergo age assessments, and every effort must be made to ensure that a child's dignity is preserved. We must also strive to create and implement safeguards to address appeals in cases of disputed results. If a child refuses to undergo any kind of age assessment, it should not be held against him/her, or prejudice the assessment or protection measures.

Ultimately, our goal should be to reduce the use of such exams and use them only as a last resort. Individually and as a profession, the best interest of the child must always be our guiding principle, and we must holistically assess each child's vulnerability and unique needs, in line with international guidelines [13,18].

4. Use Our Collective Voices

We should also urge professional medical organizations and associations such as the American Academy of Pediatrics, American Dental Association, American College of Dentists, American Board of Forensic Odontology, American College of Radiology, and the American Academy of Forensic Sciences to offer guidance to their members about all the medical, legal, and ethical issues inherent in age assessments and to help educate other stakeholders—for example, immigration judges—about common pitfalls of using imaging for age assessment.

Conflicts of Interest: The author declares no conflict of interest. The author is a paid expert medical consultant for Physicians for Human Rights' (PHR) Program on Sexual Violence in Conflict Zones, a member of PHR's asylum network and the faculty leader of Georgetown University Medical Center's Asylum Program.

References

1. Hjern, A.; Brendler-Lindqvist, M.; Norredam, M. Age assessment of young asylum seekers. *Acta Paediatr.* **2012**, *101*, 4–7. [CrossRef] [PubMed]
2. Urschler, M.; Krauskopf, A.; Widek, T.; Sorantin, E.; Ehammer, T.; Borkenstein, M.; Yen, K.; Scheurer, E. Applicability of Greulich-Pyle and Tanner-Whitehouse grading methods to MRI when assessing hand bone age in forensic age estimation: A pilot study. *Forensic Sci. Int.* **2016**, *266*, 281–288. [CrossRef] [PubMed]
3. Emmanuel, M.; Bokor, B.R. Tanner Stages. In *StatPearls*; StatPearls Publishing: Treasure Island, FL, USA, 2019. Available online: http://www.ncbi.nlm.nih.gov/books/NBK470280/ (accessed on 30 June 2019).
4. McDowell, M.A.; Fryar, C.D.; Ogden, C.L.; Flegal, K.M. *Anthropometric Reference Data for Children and Adults: United States, 2003–2006: (623932009-001)*; American Psychological Association: Washington, DC, USA, 2008. [CrossRef]
5. McDowell, M.A.; Fryar, C.D.; Ogden, C.L.; Flegal, K.M. Anthropometric reference data for children and adults: United States, 2003–2006. *Natl. Health Stat. Rep.* **2008**, *10*, 1–48.
6. Kvaal, S.I.; Haugen, M. Comparisons between skeletal and dental age assessment in unaccompanied asylum seeking children. *J. Forensic Odontostomatol.* **2017**, *2*, 109–116. [PubMed]
7. Hojreh, A.; Gamper, J.; Schmook, M.T.; Weber, M.; Prayer, D.; Herold, C.J.; Noebauer-Huhmann, I.M. Hand MRI and the Greulich-Pyle atlas in skeletal age estimation in adolescents. *Skelet. Radiol.* **2018**, *47*, 963–971. [CrossRef] [PubMed]
8. Vieth, V.; Schulz, R.; Heindel, W.; Pfeiffer, H.; Buerke, B.; Schmeling, A.; Ottow, C. Forensic age assessment by 3.0T MRI of the knee: Proposal of a new MRI classification of ossification stages. *Eur. Radiol.* **2018**, *28*, 3255–3262. [CrossRef] [PubMed]
9. The Separated Children in Europe Programme (SCEP). Position Paper on Age Assessment in the Context of Separated Children in Europe. 2012. Available online: https://www.refworld.org/pdfid/4ff535f52.pdf (accessed on 30 June 2019).
10. De Sanctis, V.; Di Maio, S.; Soliman, A.T.; Raiola, G.; Elalaily, R.; Millimaggi, G. Hand X-ray in pediatric endocrinology: Skeletal age assessment and beyond. *Indian J. Endocrinol. Metab.* **2014**, *18* (Suppl. 1), S63–S71. [CrossRef]
11. Roberts, G.J.; Parekh, S.; Petrie, A.; Lucas, V.S. Dental age assessment (DAA): A simple method for children and emerging adults. *Br. Dent. J.* **2008**, *204*, E7. [CrossRef] [PubMed]
12. Serinelli, S.; Panetta, V.; Pasqualetti, P.; Marchetti, D. Accuracy of three age determination X-ray methods on the left hand-wrist: A systematic review and meta-analysis. *Leg. Med.* **2011**, *13*, 120–133. [CrossRef]

13. Aynsley-Green, A.; Cole, T.J.; Crawley, H.; Lessof, N.; Boag, L.R.; Wallace, R.M.M. Medical, statistical, ethical and human rights considerations in the assessment of age in children and young people subject to immigration control. *Br. Med. Bull.* **2012**, *102*, 17–42. [CrossRef]
14. Malmqvist, E.; Furberg, E.; Sandman, L. Ethical aspects of medical age assessment in the asylum process: A Swedish perspective. *Int. J. Legal. Med.* **2018**, *132*, 815–823. [CrossRef] [PubMed]
15. Unaccompanied Minors and the Flores Settlement Agreement: What to Know > National Conference of State Legislatures. Available online: http://www.ncsl.org/blog/2018/10/30/unaccompanied-minors-and-the-flores-settlement-agreement-what-to-know.aspx (accessed on 30 June 2019).
16. Flores—United States District Court Central District of California. Available online: https://cliniclegal.org/sites/default/files/attachments/flores_v._reno_settlement_agreement_1.pdf (accessed on 30 June 2019).
17. Informed Consent in Decision-Making in Pediatric Practice|from the American Academy of Pediatrics|Pediatrics. Available online: https://pediatrics-aappublications-org.proxy.library.georgetown.edu/content/138/2/e20161484 (accessed on 28 June 2019).
18. United Nations High Commissioner of Refugees (UNHCR). *Inter-Agency Guiding Principles on Unaccompanied and Separated Children*; UNHCR: Geneva, Switzerland, 2004; Available online: https://www.unhcr.org/protection/children/4098b3172/inter-agency-guiding-principles-unaccompanied-separated-children.html (accessed on 20 July 2019).

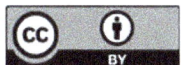

© 2019 by the author. Licensee MDPI, Basel, Switzerland. This article is an open access article distributed under the terms and conditions of the Creative Commons Attribution (CC BY) license (http://creativecommons.org/licenses/by/4.0/).

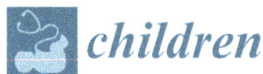

Opinion

The Rights of *Children on the Move* and the Budapest Declaration

Charles Oberg

Divisions of Global Pediatrics and Epidemiology & Community Health, University of Minnesota, 717 Delaware Street, Minneapolis, MN 55414, USA; oberg001@umn.edu

Received: 16 April 2018; Accepted: 15 May 2018; Published: 17 May 2018

Abstract: It has been estimated that more than 50,000,000 children and youth have migrated across borders or been forcibly displaced within their own country. They consist of refugees, asylum seekers, internally displaced persons (IDP), economic migrants, and exploited trafficked children. They are virtually "stateless", children deprived of the protective structures of state and family that they need and deserve and unrecognized by either their country of origin or the international community. This opinion piece starts with the personal reflections of its author on his recent work in Middle East refugee camps. It then explores the prevalence and demographics of these children and their plight. It examines the United Nation's Convention on the Rights of the Child (CRC) and other international conventions designed to protect them. It also summarizes the International Society of Social Pediatrics and Child Health (ISSOP) Budapest Declaration on the Rights, Health and Well-Being of Children and Youth on the Move as a framework for improved care and vehicle for change.

Keywords: migration; refugee; internally displaced persons (IDP); immigrant; children's rights; Budapest Declaration

1. Introduction

It has been estimated that more than 50,000,000 children have migrated across borders or been forcibly displaced within their own country [1]. This includes 28,000,000 uprooted children who are either refugees living outside their country of origin or internally displaced due to wars, violence and conflict [2]. What is even more staggering is the 75% increase in the number of child refugees between 2010 and 2015 [3].

This crisis now directly affects every continent on the globe and indirectly each and every one of us. Over the last few years, the plight of children on the move became personal. I had the opportunity to work in several refugee camps serving displaced children. The first was on the Greek island of Lesvos. I volunteered with the Boat Refugee Foundation (BRF), a Netherlands based non-governmental organization NGO. The majority of my time was spent in the notorious Moria Refugee Camp with over 4500 refugees. Based in an old army compound, the camp was defined by the steel gates, high fencing and barbwire on the perimeter with an amorphous sea of tarps and tents on the inside. It was during the winter months and a few days prior to my arrival, the weather had turned brutally cold. Over a foot of snow was followed by freezing rain. The cold and dampness penetrated to the bone. Food queues, inadequate unsanitary toilet facilities and ubiquitous garbage were the norm. More recently, I traveled with the Syrian American Refugee Society (SAMS) to provide care to Syrian refugee children in multiple locations in northern Jordan. The most were in Al Zaatari, presently the second largest refugee camp in the world with over 80,000 inhabitants.

Despite best efforts, primary care was inadequate, referrals limited or non-existent and quality shelter and nutrition hard to provide in such settings. Children spend days, weeks and months with little opportunity to play in a safe and nurturing environment. There are multiple NGO's providing assistance including UNHCR, Save the Children, Euro Relief, the Red Cross/Red Crescent and others. However, the task of providing a safe milieu to grow, thrive and play is limited. In addition, many of the children have experience and/or witnessed trauma either in their home country or on their exodus to safety and a new life. Access to mental health services is woefully limited. Almost all the children and youth had experienced trauma. Some beaten, shot, tortured, and raped and all had experienced the stress of living in unlivable conditions. The complaints were a blur of physical, mental, and spiritual aliments.

Yet there was a palpable hope that one-day things would be better with aspirations of a better future. Daily they expressed their gratitude that someone would listen as they shared the story of their journey, affirmed their worth, acknowledged their struggle and celebrated their humanity. You could see it in their eyes and their smiles that each was seeking a better life for themselves and their children. I saw no terrorist. I just saw families, children, men and women—all vulnerable and suffering.

The children I saw were just a fraction of the millions of children and youth who have been displaced from their homes due to war, conflict, natural disasters and families seeking a better life.

2. The Scope of the Problem

The problem of children displaced from their homes spans decades and will most certainly worsen in the future due to the scope of the problem and the lack of an appropriate international response. This section provides a sampling of the magnitude of the problem. It is essential to first identify that the plight of Palestinians represent the largest and longest displaced group of refugees. For seven decades the global community has closed its eyes and has ignored millions of forgotten children now living in the occupied territories of Gaza and the West Bank as well as those who been dispersed throughout the Middle East in Lebanon, Jordan, and Syria. The majority of Palestinians (3.7 million children and young people) are under the age of 25, and 40% of (2.5 million) are under the age of 18 [4]. Every decade since has experienced its own diaspora. This includes but is not limited to the exodus that started from Southeast Asia in the 1970–1980's and Somalia in the 1990's [5,6]. Since the turn of the millennium, refugees have fled the conflict and wars in Iraq, Afghanistan, and Syria. Africa has also experienced multiple displacements of children throughout the continent. Most recently the world has witnessed the persecuted Rohingya fleeing Myanmar into Bangladesh [7,8].

Children on the move also include millions of children migrating either with their families or as unaccompanied children and youth who are not fleeing war but are seeking a safer environment and opportunity for the future. Frequently labeled economic migrants, they are trying to escape poverty, exploitation, limited opportunity and frequently violence [9]. This includes the children and youth being forced into child labor or sex trafficked [10,11].

The situation has been exacerbated by a gradual shift in our response to this crisis at the national and international level. Though not uniform, we see growing intolerance and disdain translated into international policy. A growing fervor of fear and xenophobia has led to the closing of borders, stricter application of refugee and asylum criteria and increasing deportation, all of which are intended to stop the human flow seeking safety and freedom. The result is "stateless" children who are neither welcomed from their country of origin or the country where their exodus ends [12]. Do these children have rights and if so what moral obligations do we, as a global community, have in addressing their plight?

3. Children's Rights and International Protection

In 1923, Eglantyne Jebb, who witnessed and documented the devastating effects of World War I on European children, penned a *Declaration of the Rights of the Child*. She later went on to start the Save the Children dedicating her life to children displaced by tragedy and war [13]. The Declaration was subsequently adopted by the United Nations in 1952 [14].

The Declaration espoused the basic principle of civil and political as well as economic, societal and cultural rights for all children. To put the Declaration into force, the UN General Assembly passed the

UN Convention on the Rights of the Child on 20 November 1989 and has become the most universally accepted treaty in the history of the United Nation [15]. Globally every nation has signed the CRC (UN Convention on the Rights of the Child) except for the United States and South Sudan. The Convention establishes the responsibility of governments, institutions, citizens and families to ensure that the rights of the child are respected and all actions are directed toward achieving the "best interest of the child" [16].

The Convention provides a framework for the protection of children on the move. It is of particular concern that most professionals who deal with families with children are unfamiliar with the provisions of the UN Convention on the Rights of the Child (CRC). The UN CRC was the first legally binding international document to recognize the rights of the child. It provides a firm legal, moral, and ethical basis to achieve equity in response to children on the move [17].

Two other UN Conventions speak to the need for vulnerable children on the move. The first is the United Nations Convention relating to the Status of Refugees, which was adopted in 1951 and entered into force in 1954. It remains the centerpiece of international refugee protection today [18]. The second is the 1990 International Convention on the Protection of the Rights of All Migrant Workers and Members of their Families, which reiterates the principle of universal protection [19].

4. Budapest Declaration

In November 2017, the International Society of Social Pediatrics and Child Health (ISSOP) passed the *Budapest Declaration—On the Rights, Health and Well-Being of Children and Youth on the Move*. This society of international pediatricians was aware of the unprecedented global displacement of children and its perverse effects on their health and well-being [20]. The Declaration advocates for the following provisions:

- Entitles all children to the full complement of rights—regardless of their displacement status;
- Enumerates requirements for a holistic response to their physical and mental health risks and needs;
- Defines the elements of leadership for pediatricians and organizations;
- Outlines requirements for evidenced-base policies, protocols and evaluation;
- Grounds this work in a global context;
- Establishes the structure of a *Child Health Action Plan for Children and Youth on the Move*.

In addition, cognizant of violations of human rights resulting from displacement, the *Declaration* establishes the first comprehensive child rights-based blueprint for global pediatric leadership and action that integrates clinical care, systems development and public policy [21]. Specifically, in the domain of clinical care it recommends; health assessments and continuity of care should be performed in a manner that is sensitive to their cultural and ethnic origins. Specifically, an awareness that refugees and immigrant families are not a homogenous population.

Rather a heterogeneous tapestry of different cultures with different beliefs around health, wellness and approaches to care. In addition, that even within a specific region or country numerous languages, dialects and distinct ethnic backgrounds must be acknowledged as providers seek to establish trust and a meaningful healing relationship. It must take place with informed consent and include participation in physical and mental health care decision making. In addition, professionals working with children should be trained in cultural and linguistic competency and how to work with interpreters.

Finally, care delivery must incorporate a trauma-informed approach to care. Trauma-informed approaches must assure that the care delivered is aware and sensitive to past traumas that have occurred in the child's home country, during their journey and in the new location that they have arrived. All efforts must be made to not re-traumatize the family or children in the administration of care. It must also establish therapeutic approaches that are developmentally appropriate for the children and youth who are being served with ancillary strategies and complementary approaches that promote healing. Health systems must recognize the physical and mental vulnerabilities across the age span including pregnant women newborns, children, adolescents and young adults.

In addition, the needs of children with disabilities must also be addressed. Service delivery systems for these children and youth, even in countries with well-established health systems, must address the fragmentation and barriers to optimal care.

An essential element of new policies is that every nation state should advance *Health in all Policies* with a commitment to global public heath that advances equity for all within their borders [22]. States parties should be held accountable for their actions to children and youth on the move within their boundaries to ensure the full implementation of the rights articulated in the CRC, and this accountability should be addressed in their periodic reports to the Committee on the Rights of the Child. As of May 2018, fifteen International Pediatric Professional Associations have endorsed the Budapest Declaration representing pediatricians from North and South America, Europe, Asia and Australia.

5. Conclusion

Pediatricians and all professionals dedicated to the care of children have critical roles to play in response to the unprecedented global displacement of children. Pediatric leadership is essential and will consist of clearly delineating roles and responsibilities for engagement with other global organizations seeking change. This must include cooperation with key partners such as the UN Childen's Fund (UNICEF), the World Health Organization (WHO) and the UN High Commissioner for Refugees (UNHCR). It will also include participation in a larger coalition of other NGO's whose goals align including the International Organization for Migration (IOM), Save the Children, and Initiative for Child Rights in the Global Compact. As the world seeks to close international borders and to implement travel bans I make a plea for benevolence and tolerance. We must find policy solutions and concrete programmatic change to address the needs of children and youth on the move. To that end ISSOP has formulated a *Child Health Action Plan for Children and Youth on the Move* and has convened a workgroup to undertake its implementation. It presently consists of twenty-five child health professionals from fifteen countries. Together with other professional organizations and NGO's an effort will be made to affect positive change. The effort will attempt to shift the global response from restricting access to expansion and openness. In the end let us remember that our kindness will make us safer than fear. This effort is part of a larger global awareness. Presently, the United Nations has undertaken a dialogue and initiated negotiations concerning Global Compact on Refugees and Migrants. It is possible that states are awakening to the particular vulnerabilities of children and youth on the move [23].

Conflicts of Interest: The author declares no conflict of interest.

References

1. *Uprooted-The Growing Crisis for Refugee and Migrant Children*; UNICEF: New York, NY, USA, 2016; p. 3.
2. *Children on the Move: Key Facts & Figures Data Brief*; UNICEF: New York, NY, USA, 2018; p. 2.
3. *Uprooted-The Growing Crisis for Refugee and Migrant Children*; UNICEF: New York, NY, USA, 2016; p. 1.
4. *The Situation of Palestinian Children in the Occupied Palestinian Territory, Jordan, Syria and Lebanon*; UNICEF Regional Office for the MENA: Amman, Jordan, 2011; p. 3.
5. Gordan, L.W. Southeast Asian Refugee Migration to the United States. In *Center for Migration Studies Special Issues*; John Wiley and Sons: Hoboken, NJ, USA, 1987; Volume 5, p. 153.
6. Rutledge, D. *The Somali Diaspora—A Journey Away*; University of Minnesota Press: Minneapolis, MN, USA, 2008.
7. UNHCR R Middle East and North Africa Civil Society Network for Displacement. Available online: http://www.unhcr.org/en-us/middle-east-and-north-africa.html (accessed on 11 April 2018).
8. JRP for Rohingya Humanitarian Crisis-March–December 2018. Available online: https://www.unocha.org/rohingya-refugee-crisis (accessed on 11 April 2018).
9. *International Migration Report 2017: Highlights (ST/ESA/SER.A/404)*; United Nations Department of Economic and Social Affairs, Population Division: New York, NY, USA, 2017.

10. Leinberger, A.; Parker, D.L.; Oberg, C.N. Child labor, gender & health. *Public Health Reports* **2005**, *120*, 642–647.
11. *Every Child Counts-New Global Estimates on Child Labour*; International Labour Office: Geneva, Switzerland, 2002.
12. Bhabha, J. Arendt's Children-Do today's children have a right to have rights? *Hum. Rights Q.* **2009**, *31*, 410–451. [CrossRef]
13. Mower, A.G. *The Convention on the Rights of the Child—International Law Support for Children*; Greenwood Press: Westport, CT, USA, 1997; p. 11.
14. LeBlanc, L.J. *The Convention on the Rights of the Child—United Nations Lawmaking on Human Rights*; University of Nebraska Press: Lincoln, NE, USA, 1995; p. 15.
15. Oberg, C.N. Embracing international children's rights-From principle to practice. *Clin. Pediatr.* **2012**, *5*, 619–624. [CrossRef] [PubMed]
16. Dupont, L.; Foley, J.; Gagliardi, A. *Raising Children with Roots, Rights and Responsibilities—Celebrating the UN Convention on the Rights of the Child*; The Human Rights Resource Center: Minneapolis, MN, USA, 1999.
17. Goldhagen, J. Children's rights and the United Nations Convention on the Rights of the Child. *Pediatrics* **2003**, *112*, 742–745. [PubMed]
18. Convention and Protocol relating to the Status of Refugees, United Nations High Commissioner for Refugees, Geneva, December 2010. Available online: http://www.unhcr.org/en-us/protection/basic/3b66c2aa10/convention-protocol-relating-status-refugees.html (accessed on 10 April 2018).
19. Blitz, B.K. Neither Seen nor Heard-Compound Deprivation among Stateless Children. In *Children without a State-A Global Human Rights Challenge*; Bhabha, J., Ed.; MIT Press: Cambridge, MA, USA, 2011; p. 46.
20. ISSOP Migration Working Group. ISSOP Position Statement on Migrant Health. *Child Care Health Dev.* **2018**, *44*, 161–170.
21. Goldhagen, J.L.; Kadir, A.; Fouad, F.M.; Spencer, N.J.; Raman, S. The Budapest Declaration for children and youth on the move. *Lancet Child Adolesc. Health* **2018**, *2*, 164–165. [CrossRef]
22. Ministry of Social Affairs and Health, Finland and World Health Organization. Health in All Policies-Helsinki Statement: Framework for Country Action 2014. Available online: http://www.ngos4healthpromotion.net/wordpressa4hp/wp-content/uploads/2016/11/helsinki.pdf (accessed on 15 May 2018).
23. United Nations Global Compact on Refugees. Available online: https://refugeesmigrants.un.org/refugees-compact (accessed on 26 April 2018).

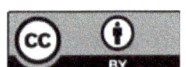

© 2018 by the author. Licensee MDPI, Basel, Switzerland. This article is an open access article distributed under the terms and conditions of the Creative Commons Attribution (CC BY) license (http://creativecommons.org/licenses/by/4.0/).

MDPI
St. Alban-Anlage 66
4052 Basel
Switzerland
Tel. +41 61 683 77 34
Fax +41 61 302 89 18
www.mdpi.com

Children Editorial Office
E-mail: children@mdpi.com
www.mdpi.com/journal/children

www.ingramcontent.com/pod-product-compliance
Lightning Source LLC
LaVergne TN
LVHW071956080526
838202LV00064B/6765